Integrative Approaches to Supervision

of related interest

Creative Supervision
The Use of Expressive Arts Methods in Supervision and Self-Supervision
Mooli Lahad
ISBN 1 85302 828 2

Systemic Supervision
A Portable Guide for Supervision Training
Gill Gorell Barnes and Gwynneth Down
ISBN 1 85302 853 3

Advocacy, Counselling and Mediation in Casework
Processes of Empowerment
Edited by Yvonne Joan Craig
ISBN 1 85302 564 X

Mediation in Context
Edited by Marian Liebmann
ISBN 1 85302 618 2

Good Practice in Supervision
Statutory and Voluntary Organisations
Edited by Jacki Pritchard
ISBN 1 85302 279 9
Good Practice in Social Work Series 2

Staff Supervision in a Turbulent Environment
Managing Process and Task in Front-line Services
Lynette Hughes and Paul Pengelly
ISBN 1 85302 327 2

Integrative Approaches to Supervision

Edited by Michael Carroll
and Margaret Tholstrup

Jessica Kingsley Publishers
London and Philadelphia

First published in the United Kingdom in 2001 by
Jessica Kingsley Publishers
116 Pentonville Road
London N1 9JB, UK
and
400 Market Street, Suite 400
Philadelphia, PA 19106, USA

www.jkp.com

Digitally printed since 2004

Library of Congress Cataloging in Publication Data
A CIP catalog record for this book is available from the Library of Congress

British Library Cataloguing in Publication Data
A CIP catalogue record for this book is available from the British Library

ISBN-13: 978 1 84985 206 7
ISBN-10: 1 84985 206 5

Contents

Figures and Tables

Acknowledgements

We would like to dedicate this book to the British Association for Supervision Practice and Research (BASPR) committee and participants for providing us with the background and content.

Michael would like to include in the dedications Mary and Gary McMahon in Brisbane; Dianne and Kevin Hawken in Auckland; John and Sarah Kidd in Christchurch; and Philip McConkey from Palmerston North who made visiting Australia and New Zealand an experience of a lifetime.

Margaret would like to include in the dedications Hubert Lacey for first introducing her to the eating disorders field; her supervision consultation group for their many years of supporting and challenging her as she developed as a supervisor; and her patient and devoted husband John, without whose love and care none of this would be possible.

Introduction

The British Association for Supervision Research and Practice (BASPR) has now been in existence for nine years. To call it an 'association' is probably a bit beyond its stature: it is more like a 'virtual association'. Its organising committee of five supervisors arranges a supervision conference each year. Their aim is to provide a meeting place for supervisors and supervisees to network and discuss the supervisory issues of the day. For each annual conference they set the theme, arrange keynote addresses and workshops pertinent to the theme and mailshot BASPR's large database of names for participants. These conferences have been both national and international and have attracted participants and presenters from the US, mainland Europe, New Zealand as well as Britain and Ireland. It is the only British forum we know of where supervisors, from all orientations and walks of life, gather to discuss and dialogue about contemporary supervisory issues and concerns.

Each year, after each conference, the organising committee meets and reminisces about the wealth of the presentations, the richness of the group, the experience and expertise which is so obvious in all those attending and how fortunate we are to have such depth and breadth to British supervision. Each year the committee says they wish someone would publish the keynote addresses and workshops, which they believe deserve a wider audience. Each year life intervenes and the conference material never sees the published light of day. There is good news: at last a change and for the first time steps have been taken to gather the 1999 conference programme into a publication. The title of the 1999 conference, 'Integrative Approaches to Supervision', has been kept and becomes the title of the proceedings. The editors have also gone slightly beyond the 1999 conference to include a few additions: Michael Carroll's keynote address at the 1998 conference on the spirituality of supervision, as well as papers by John Towler on sub-personalities in supervision and Joanna Beazley Richards and Gary Leonard on liability issues for supervisors.

Since BASPR's inception nine years ago supervision theory research and practice has developed by leaps and bounds in Britain and the British supervisory scene quite rightly prides itself on the quality of its practice. The titles of the chapters in this publication attest to this: in them supervision is allied to such diverse issues as spirituality, life stages, organisations, primary health care, eating disorders, mental health, race, culture, personality, Jungian typology, narrative approaches, the law and finally future directions for the profession in the new millennium.

The book chapters do not appear in the order in which the subjects were presented at the conference. Instead the editors have divided them into three parts for coherence and focus: Part 1 comprises six chapters around the theme of Models and Frameworks of Intergrative Supervision. Part 2 connects supervision to three areas: mental heath, primary health care and people with eating disorders. The final set of chapters, Part 3, centre on supervision and specific issues such as race and culture, personality types, researching theraputic practice, complaints and litigation, finishing with some thoughts on challenges facing supervision in the new millennium.

The diversity as shown here indicates how important supervision has become in the professional life of British mental health. From the doing has come the research, the theories, the practice and the skills of supervision. These are fed back into the practice, creating an experiential learning wheel of doing, reflecting, learning and applying.

The chapters here are written in that vein: all of them originated as presentations and were spoken to their audiences. In editing this book the editors did not want to lose that richness and the impact of that mode of delivery. We wanted authors to edit their own written work for publication and thereby retain the strengths of both the spoken and the written word. Aware that asking for both could result in getting neither to an acceptable level, we consider that the authors have done a fine job. For this we thank them.

Our thanks also to the BASPR committee (Brigid Proctor, Maria Gilbert, Michael Carroll, Paul Hitchings and Terri Spy) who have toiled over the past nine years to arrange and plan each conference and who have encouraged this book. Without them there would be no BASPR, no BASPR conference and no publication.

Michael Carroll
Margaret Tholstrup

Note

The British Association for Counseling is now the British Association for Counseling and Psychotherapy.

PART 1

Models and Frameworks of Integrative Supervision

Chapter 1

The Cyclical Model of Supervision

A Container for Creativity and Chaos

Val Wosket and Steve Page

It has been suggested that we need a new term for the activity we call 'supervision', yet the word itself seems adequately to reflect the functions and tasks ascribed to that role. The dictionary definition describes a supervisor as an 'overseer', a word that conveys a sense of taking the broader view. A supervisor is someone who can cast a detached yet concerned and compassionate eye over the landscape of counselling practice and, in so doing, can often pick out the detail that hovers at the supervisee's peripheral vision and which is not always clearly seen.

Perhaps the suggestions that arise for a change of name reflect a growing recognition of the complexity of the supervisory tasks and process. Maybe some commentators feel that we need a more grandiose title to accompany the increased sophistication of the role that is now described and analysed at great length in the growing literature on supervision. The burgeoning of models and approaches to supervision that has occurred over the last decade can be greeted with some alarm. Even now, novel approaches to supervision are appearing specifically designed to accompany the newer counselling models of brief and solution focused therapy (O'Connell and Jones 1997; Selekman and Todd 1995). The alarm is about the danger that supervision, like counselling and psychotherapy, may come to suffer from an over-proliferation of models, schools and approaches. As Goldfried and Pradawer (1982) have observed there indeed 'comes a time when one needs to question where fruitful diversity ends and where chaos begins' (p.3). A genuine hazard related to the proliferation of supervision models is that an over-emphasis on techniques and set procedures will ensue in which simplicity, humanity and spontaneity are elbowed out as the unseemly bedfellows of carefully planned interventionist strategies. The velocity with which new models of supervision are bursting forth suggests it might be a helpful time to pause, review and assess where we are at this stage in the growth and development of supervision. This steady stream may soon turn into an avalanche from which it may become increasingly difficult to dig our way out and gain a clear view of key landmarks in the surrounding landscape. Some landmark questions relating to the topic that have immediate currency might be:

- why have a model of supervision?
- how, if at all, is a model of supervision better than no model?
- does a supervision training course require a core model?
- what are the tasks and purposes of a supervision model?
- what are the disadvantages and dangers of using a supervision model and how might they best be avoided?

This chapter will attempt to offer a response to some of these fundamental questions. As a prelude to so doing, it is useful to be clear about what we mean by supervision in the UK as opposed, say, to what is usually meant by supervision in the US. In America, supervision is considered to be a necessity for trainees and interns and, not surprisingly therefore, has a strong educational component. For licensed professionals supervision is variously viewed, depending on perspective and circumstance, as lying somewhere between an impractical luxury and a remedial necessity when things go wrong (Carr 1994). And while training for supervisors is now well established in this country, in the US specialist training for supervisors it is not widely seen as necessary. Indeed, there have been suggestions that incentives may be needed to encourage would-be supervisors to attend training courses. Kaslow (1986) is one of the few American writers who advocates training for supervisors working in educational institutions. Yet in order to get them to attend training events she suggests (and this seems to be a serious suggestion) that they are offered perks in the form of enhanced 'library privileges, and/or free parking on busy campuses' (p.7).

In Britain, though it is beginning to be challenged in some quarters (Feltham 1999; 2000), supervision is still generally viewed as a career-long requirement for practising counsellors and psychotherapists. The attitude that most therapists in the UK today hold towards supervision was summed up recently by one of our first year counselling students. On her end of year course evaluation form she highlighted supervision, which she had never encountered before, as one of the best aspects of the course and described it as 'a luxurious necessity'. In this chapter we are taking the view of supervision, arguably predominant in the UK, that it is a necessary part of ongoing professional development for the counselling practitioner.

In setting out our own position, we believe that we need to be able to account for how we work as supervisors. We should be prepared to give a considered rationale for this to our supervisees in the same way that we believe we have an obligation to our counselling clients to de-mystify the therapeutic process for them as far as is possible. We hope to argue that becoming thoroughly grounded in a best-fit model of supervision goes a long way towards achieving such accountability.

So, why *do* we think we need a model of supervision? As counsellors we are required to work within our known areas of competence. We adopt assessment and intake procedures that allow us the space to reflect on whether we have the skills, experience and personal aptitude to help particular clients with their specific areas of difficulty. As supervisors we do not generally have the opportunity to engage with such an extended reflexive self-assessment process. We are normally obliged to respond in the moment to whatever our supervisees bring – whether or not it is something we have come across before or worked with ourselves. Usually we will have no idea about what our supervisees might serve up to us before we sit down with them to listen to their dilemmas. A couple of recent examples of encountering the unexpected within my own experience [Val] as a supervisor and supervisee illustrate the point:

> My supervisee tells me that she has recently been on a religious pilgrimage. One of her clients is aware of this and in the session when she next sees him after her return, he asks her if they can hold hands and pray together. My supervisee tells her client that she needs to think about this before making a response and she brings the dilemma to me. It is one I have never faced myself.

> I take to my own supervisor my work with a client who is beginning to disclose experiences of extreme sadistic childhood abuse, including sexual, psychological and physical torture. My supervisor tells me that this is the worst case of abuse she has heard of and that she has never dealt with anything like it herself.

How does the supervisor begin to know how to respond to such situations? Borders (1992) makes the simple but crucial point that in making the transition from counsellor to supervisor, the becoming-supervisor needs to make a cognitive shift from thinking like a counsellor to thinking like a supervisor. This involves, primarily, a shift in focus from the client to the counsellor. She suggests that supervisors who think like supervisors rather than like counsellors need to 'ask themselves "How can I intervene so that this counsellor will be more effective with current and future clients?"' (p.138). Supervisors who fail to make this shift are more likely to approach sessions 'well prepared to tell the counsellor what they would do with this client' (p.137). As Borders suggests, the likely result then is that 'supervisees become surrogate counselors who [merely] carry out supervisors' plans for counseling' (p.137).

Having a model of counselling supervision can help the supervisor answer the question 'How can I intervene so that this counsellor will be more effective with current and future clients?' A model of supervision can provide both a container for holding and a process for working with the unknown and the unexpected. A supervision model should, above all else, help release power in the supervisee to enable the clients – rather than first and foremost empower the supervisor. Thus the cyclical model of supervision, which is discussed below, is intended to promote the autonomy of supervisees more than it is to educate them. The model provides a container that can hold the counsellor in and to their task, even when the supervisee might be dealing with something their supervisor has not encountered or even imagined – and therefore may well *not* be able to educate the supervisee about.

Do supervision training courses need a core model of supervision? The counselling arena has recently hosted a vigorous debate between those who support a core model of counselling for training courses and those who question the necessity of a core model (Connor 1994; Dryden, Horton and Mearns 1995; Feltham 1995; 1996; 1997; 1999; Horton 1996; Wheeler 1998). The time may now be ripe to take this debate into the supervision arena, given the recent rapid increase in training courses in supervision in Britain. Some of the arguments in favour of core models in supervision training might be placed under the following headings.

1. *Providing knowledge and security.* When people are learning about counselling or supervision they require a reasonable amount of certainty and consistency in order to be able to invoke creativity and risk taking. A core model can provide the beginning supervisor with a clear idea of the operation of the supervision process and a sound repertoire of enabling interventions. From a secure base provided by a core model trainee supervisors can then further refine and develop their own styles of supervision in response to additional influences such as the needs of specific counsellor and client populations and the requirements of different organisational contexts.

2. *Establishing a reliable framework.* Having a reliable and familiar framework that is well known and integrated can encourage innovation and flexibility while helping to contain the high levels of anxiety to which a trainee supervisor can succumb as they make the transition from counsellor to supervisor. The supervisor who is learning to venture out on his or her own has, in the core model, a safe and certain 'parent' to return to and look back upon when a steadying presence is needed. Beginning supervisors will inevitably lose their footing on occasion and need to know that when this happens they can fall back on and be guided by a tried and trusted model.

3. *Providing way markers.* Frank (1989, p.109) has argued that the 'rationale and ritual' of a theory or model of therapy can provide a foundation that gives counselling trainees their initial impetus, confidence and direction. Similarly, a core model of supervision provides the necessary way markers to help a beginning supervisor find a set route through the complex maze that is the supervision process until experience comes to provide a more innate sense of direction.

4. *Averting the danger of random eclecticism.* Corey, Corey and Callanan (1993, p.216) have likened the counsellor who operates without an explicit core theoretical rationale to the pilot who attempts to fly a plane without instruments or a map. The same analogy translates to supervision where initial allegiance to a clearly differentiated and sufficiently comprehensive core model gives the novice supervisor a range of systematic operating procedures. This in turn lessens the likelihood that he or she will engage in undisciplined manoeuvres, which may result in the unfortunate supervisee ricocheting from the effects of one haphazard intervention after another. Supervisors who have not subjected themselves to the disciplined study of one extended philosophy and methodology of supervision are in danger of spewing forth a random application of techniques. Such behaviour is more than likely driven by desperate efforts to get the supervisee, and maybe their client, somewhere by the end of the session at any cost.

5. *Building confidence.* Thorough study and practice of a model of supervision can build confidence in that a model is something tangible to which the trainee can attribute successful interventions and thereby start to build up a useful bank of precedents that can be referred to in future work. Allegiance to a model can help the supervisor maintain equilibrium and a sense of competence in the face of difficult challenges. Just as an important part of learning to be an effective counsellor is learning to trust the therapeutic process, so supervisors need to have a supervision process they can adhere to and trust when the work with supervisees becomes turbulent or is becalmed.

6. *Managing doubts and insecurities.* During stressful periods supervisors, in particular perhaps when they are starting out, may suffer from the same doubts, anxieties and insecurities manifested by their supervisees. A sound core model of supervision can provide a lifebelt that keeps the supervisor afloat and prevents him or her being dragged under by the difficulties and dilemmas brought by supervisees. At times it may only be the overlay of training and a clear conceptualisation of the supervision process and tasks that marks a difference between the

supervisor and his or her supervisees. Lewin (1996) has commented that 'therapists gain security from their theoretical notions, as from a fetish or a teddy bear, that helps them stay organised and so be effective' (p.26). The same may well be true for supervisors. When a supervision model is well articulated and integrated it encourages the supervisor to work in a thoughtful and supervisee-responsive manner. She or he will thereby begin to trust that what they are providing is of benefit even when the work is slow and halting and the supervisee's client appears to be making little progress. Without the security of a sound model to frame and guide the process the supervisor is in some danger of going for the quick fix approach. This in turn may easily slide into advice giving or teaching in which the supervisor becomes a substitute counsellor and disenfranchises their supervisees of their own autonomous decisions.

7. *Providing techniques and intervention strategies.* Hobson (1985) has commented that 'in the earlier stages of learning a trainee usually needs a core model with definite techniques. There is an urgent need to elucidate some basic principles which, later, can be questioned, modified, or rejected' (p.209). While he is writing here about counselling trainees his words apply equally to those learning about how to be supervisors. As trainees move from being novice supervisees to seasoned practitioners the scaffolding of the core model will be less relied upon and may to a large degree be dismantled. Rather than being at the forefront of the work the model will certainly recede into the background where it will carry the function of providing a loose organising framework rather than a set procedure to be slavishly adhered to at all times.

If these can be said to be some of the advantages of a core supervision model, what about disadvantages and drawbacks? The main disadvantage, as we see it, of developing strict allegiance to a core supervision model is that it can become a strait jacket for practitioners that forces them into certain fixed postures and poses that can feel unnatural or constricting, or which stifle innovation and discovery. Supervisees, too, can be subjected to interventions prescribed by the model without due consideration being given to individual needs and differences. There is an essential tension for those who educate supervisors. It is how to promote healthy and creative scepticism in their trainees while delivering a model of supervision that promotes sufficient confidence and personal conviction to enable novice supervisors to embark on the daunting journey of accompanying and assisting counsellors who are often in difficulty with their clients.

A further danger attending over-reliance on a model of supervision is that the supervisor may miss what the model does not encompass. By their very nature models are formed by establishing boundaries. While a model of supervision, as is argued more fully later in this chapter, can be a container for creativity and chaos, it may also exclude or eliminate that which it is not designed to contain. While models can give focus and direction and guide the supervisor's interventions, they may also foreclose on what appears inconsistent with the model and suppress conflicting approaches or preferences.

Paradoxically, the supervisor who uses a model effectively needs to have the ability and willingness to abandon the model when the supervision work requires an unusual or unfamiliar response. For instance, one stage of the cyclical model, as we shall see, is concerned with encouraging the supervisee to prepare carefully for supervision by bringing a focus for the work. Yet on occasion it may be crucial that the supervisee who is struggling to find a focus is encouraged to bring that struggle in order to work on it with their supervisor. The area of occlusion may then become the focus of the supervision.

We want, now, to look more specifically at our cyclical model of counsellor supervision providing 'a container for creativity and chaos'. This title results from our wish to bring together the cyclical model and the work we have been doing since that model was first published in 1994. Val has been researching the theme of 'the therapeutic use of self' in counselling, research and supervision (Wosket 1999). In parallel I [Steve] have been exploring how we, as practitioners, deal with the darker aspects of ourselves and the role, using the Jungian concept of 'shadow' (Page 1999a). In our different but complementary ways we have both been exploring the theme of the person who is the counsellor: how their 'personhood' can at times inform and add the essential spark of humanity to the relationship with their clients and therefore to the therapeutic process. Yet at other times some aspect of themselves can cause them to stumble in this relationship, losing sight of their role as a practitioner and undermining the therapeutic endeavour. This is a tension that all therapeutic practitioners face – the tension between operating within the appropriate parameters of the role on the one hand and being authentic in their relationship with their clients on the other. This is not a static tension, but one that shifts and changes as the practitioner shifts and moves in their development. In this context we agree with Wilkins (1997) that personal and professional development cannot be separated into discrete strands so we have to think about development as an inclusive process. We are therefore encompassing these ideas while exploring our model as an example of an integrative approach to supervision (Wosket 2000). We do this through the notion of our model as a container, with chaos and creativity as aspects of what it tries to contain.

To try to get hold of the nature of the potential chaos within a supervision session two perspectives on the process of practitioner development will be considered. The first comes from the work of Skovholt and Rønnestad (1995) in which they looked at stages of development from pre-training through to pre-retirement, by interviewing 100 practitioners across this range.

Table 1.1: Stages in the evolution of the practitioner. Adapted from Skovholt and Rønnestad (1995)
The 'learning' phase • Starting training • Imitation of experts • Consolidation
The 'unlearning' (or 'integrating') phase • Exploration • Integration • Individuation

They propose eight stages, but in this summary the pre-training and the pre-retirement stages are omitted and the middle six are grouped into two broad bands. The first we have called the 'learning phase', during which the focus is upon seeking to learn the role of counsellor or therapist through training, practice and emulation of more experienced practitioners. The authors suggest that this typically lasts from initial training through to a few years post qualification. The second phase, which we have termed the 'unlearning phase', involves the process of integrating the learnt role with personal qualities and developing an authentic style of one's own. This takes the next 30 years or more!

Alongside this we want to put the practitioner's relationship with their shadow. The term 'shadow' is being used in an essentially Jungian (Jung 1959) way: describing those aspects of self that are currently and consistently out of conscious awareness and have the potential to be harmful in some way. This is both the personal shadow, and also the role shadow that is developed as the practitioner learns the role of counsellor or therapist.

> One example of my personal shadow is a tendency to feel undue guilt. It undoubtedly comes from my Roman Catholic upbringing and leaves me vulnerable to feeling unrealistically responsible for events over which I have little

> or no influence. It is of my shadow in that although I know of it and am learning more about this aspect of myself nevertheless on occasions it does influence my thoughts, feelings and actions without my realising this at the time. Not surprisingly I have to attend to this in my own supervision because it can quite easily get tangled up with my work as a counsellor, and as a supervisor.

'Role shadow' is a term used to describe the way we seem to banish aspects of ourselves when becoming counsellors because they don't fit our initial view of the role.

> Examples of my role shadow include my bluntness, sense of the ridiculous, capacity for making mischief and impatience. These are all attributes that I am generally willing to express in my personal relationships, but tend to suppress when I am working, particularly with clients. I have noticed that as I have gained in experience so it has become more frequent that I express these aspects of myself in relationships with clients, but only when a good level of trust and intimacy has developed between us. I am rather intrigued by this notion of role shadow and am inclined to think that its development is an unavoidable process for all but those who are highly self-aware. Not least because the limitations imposed by the learnt role act as one of the containers or safety devices for personal shadow material. (Page 1999a)

Building on the work of the two Roberts, Johnson (1991) and Bly (1988), a six-stage model for our relationship with our shadow has been proposed. This moves from formation through denial, recognition, confrontation, and incorporation to a point when it becomes possible to be guided by our shadow (Page 1999a). At any one time each of us is at various points along this path with different aspects of ourselves.

By now the potential for chaos is hopefully becoming apparent. In the supervision session we have counsellors who are involved in a complex developmental process that includes their personal life journey, their professional role and the interaction between the two. They are trying, presumably with integrity and commitment, to work with clients in an effectively therapeutic manner. They come to supervision where they and their supervisor attempt to engage in a dialogue in order to facilitate the counsellor's work with their clients. The supervisor is there to attend to the work with the client in parallel with endeavouring to facilitate the development of their supervisee. In addition the supervisor also has his or her own unaware or unconscious dynamics at work, stemming from their unresolved personal shadow and the role shadow formed when becoming a supervisor. To seek out examples of our own supervisor role shadow we might usefully look at our beliefs about being a good supervisor and the implicit prohibitions they contain. For example, we believe that supervisors should be supportive and encouraging, looking for the positives in what the supervisee is bringing. This is rooted in a painful experience one of us [Steve] had with a supervisor.

> This supervisor, I felt, was at times unduly harsh in his criticism and I would sometimes leave supervision feeling thoroughly despondent about my practice. In retrospect, I believe that as a result of this experience I have tended to deny my own negative critic when acting as a supervisor. As a result this has become part of my supervisor role shadow which I had to confront when faced with a supervisee some aspects of whose practice were, in my view, appalling. I eventually had to tell them that I seriously doubted their suitability for the role, asked them to cease practising and brought our supervisory relationship to an end. This caused me considerable anguish at the time.

This, then, is one way of describing the potential chaos within the supervision session. Fortunately this is not the whole picture by any means, for alongside, and indeed one might argue from within, the chaos is the potential for creativity. When we talk of creativity in the context of supervision we are thinking of the stray feeling, insight or image that offers a way forward or a new perspective, or a shift of feeling that indicates some movement in the emotional field. It is generally unexpected when it does arise; it cannot be sought but has simply to be allowed to happen and noticed as it does. This association between chaos and creativity is not limited to supervision: there are many instances across the range of human experience where chaos and destructiveness are witnessed hand-in-hand with creativity and healing.

Supervisors can define their task as:

- assisting in containing the potential destructiveness or chaos of the practitioner
- facilitating the release of creative potential to enhance the therapeutic work
- facilitating the practitioner's development.

As supervisors, we need to be willing to head towards the chaos, to deliberately seek it out, believing that it is in so doing that we open up the opportunity for creativity to emerge. If we play safe or don't undertake the task wholeheartedly the results are likely to be decidedly pedestrian.

> I [Steve] have started to learn to sail over recent months. One of the greatest surprises has been discovering that it is possible to go fast by heading toward the wind! Not directly into it but about 15 or 20 degrees either side. In comparison sailing with the wind behind you is slower and can become a little tedious – unless the wind is really blowing or you have a spinnaker of course! I think that as supervisors we do well to head as close to the wind as possible, tacking as and when necessary.

Turning now to the cyclical model[1], illustrated in Figure 1.1, we want to consider how it can be a vehicle for this task. At the heart of the model is the section that we entitle 'space'. It is here, in the centre of the work, that there is the greatest opportunity for chaos and creativity to co-exist. It is here that, as the supervisor, we can relax and allow ourselves not to know what is taking place, not know where the dialogue is taking us, to follow our instincts, intuitions, interests and to encourage the supervisee to do the same. This is the primordial soup or the alchemist's mixture that is so essential for the creative process. The slightly mysterious notion of alchemy is introduced because there is, at times, a mysterious element to what takes place here.

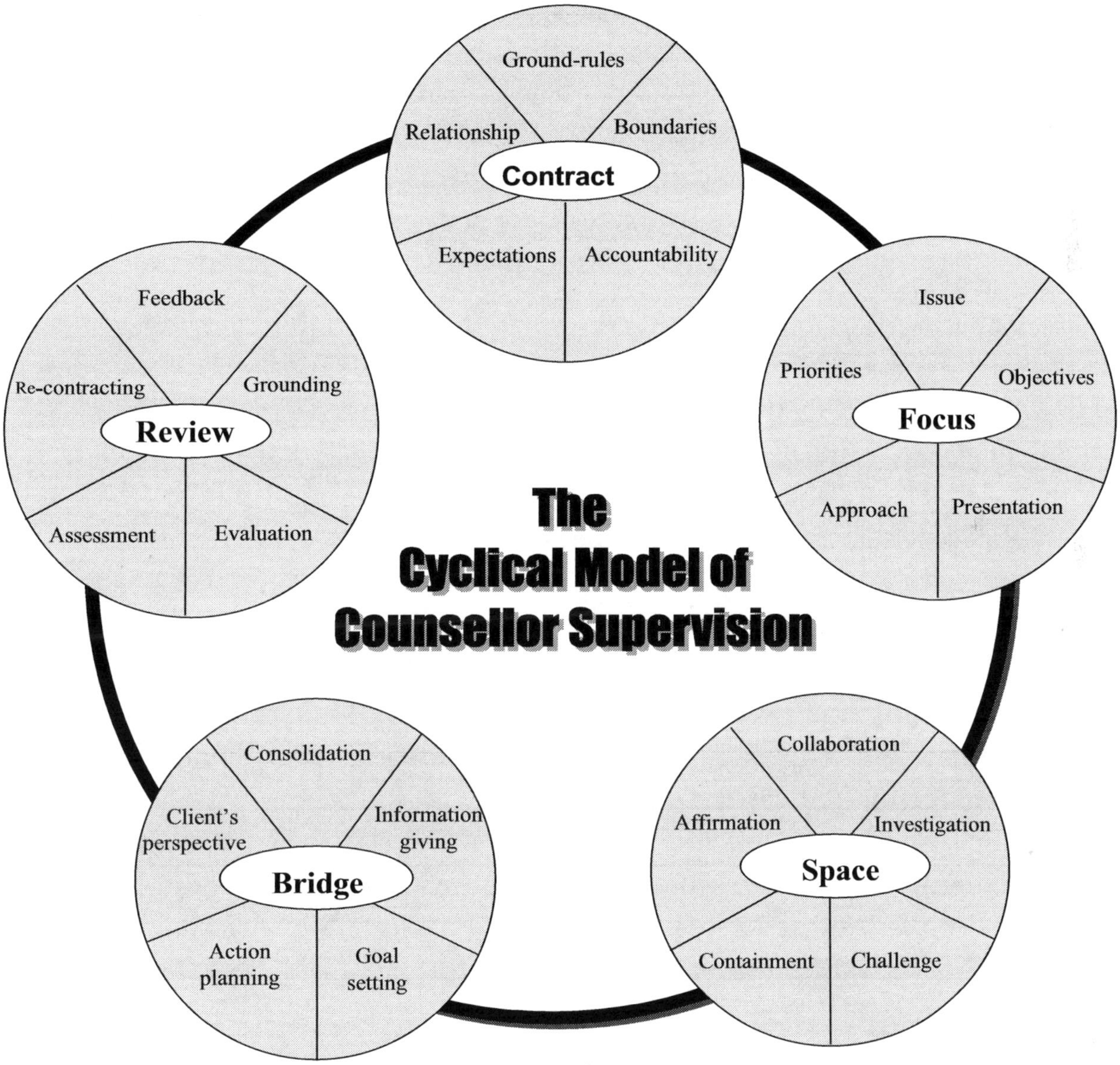

Figure 1.1: The cyclical model of counsellor supervision. This version of the model, copyright Page and Wosket (2001), was first published in poster form at the British Association for Counselling Research Conference, Leeds (UK) in 1999 (Page 1999b).

This can be illustrated with a relatively everyday example from a supervision group.

> One of the counsellors in the group presented their work with a particular client. This was a client who was deeply anguished by the death of her child. The counsellor told of this and how difficult it was for her to know how to work with this client, whom she felt was really struggling to face this experience, seemingly stuck in a deeply desperate state. The counsellor was torn between simply being with the client and following her lead and wanting to encourage her explicitly to focus upon her loss. The counsellor talked about the impact of this work on her and was herself very upset as she talked of the client. The whole group was palpably moved listening to this story. By the end of the presentation those involved in the group felt able to do little other than offer human support to the counsellor, encourage her to stay with the task and bear witness to the authenticity of what she had presented. At the next meeting of the supervision group this counsellor reported how the client had been transformed next time she saw her (transformation being the goal of alchemy). The client was lively, direct in the way she related, able to talk more freely and displayed all the hallmarks of someone moving well through a grieving process.

In one way there is nothing remarkable in this story, although it was powerful to live through. We cannot be sure that what took place in supervision had anything to do with the change in the client, but such shifts happen too frequently for me to want to deny any connection. We can give this phenomenon a name – perhaps it is a form of what we call 'parallel process' – or be comfortable just thinking of it as an empirical mystery and being glad that it happens.

Returning to 'space,' we propose that it is here that the creativity can emerge, through reflection and exploration. But for this to occur the supervisee and supervisor need to feel safe, to feel contained or held. It is hard to be creative when feeling anxious or unsafe. Notice that both supervisee and supervisor need to feel safe. The supervisor may, through the qualities they offer, provide much of this sense of safety for the supervisee. Indeed this is the Winnicottian image of supervision that Hawkins and Shohet (1989) describe: the supervisor as symbolic father providing the sense of security for the counsellor (symbolic mother) who in turn provides the security for the client (symbolic child). But if the supervisory *relationship* is to be truly creative it is not enough for the supervisee to feel secure: the supervisor needs to feel safe also.

At this point we want to start to build a new pictorial representation of our model which is illustrated in Figure 1.2. This new picture looks at the model specifically as a means of providing containment, with reference to supervisor and supervisee.

With this picture in mind the next stage to consider is the 'bridge', when attention turns to the implications of what has been explored for the next and subsequent meetings between counsellor and client. Having this as a clearly defined task means that during the exploration in the 'space' it is possible to set these issues of application to one side. This has an inevitable containing effect – to set something down knowing that there will be an opportunity to pick it up later means that we don't have to be thinking about it, or worrying about it. It is a bit like having a 'to do' list in your diary or a shopping list on the fridge door. As supervisors we can let go, for a while, of our sense of shared responsibility to consider what the counsellor is going to do as a consequence of our discussions.

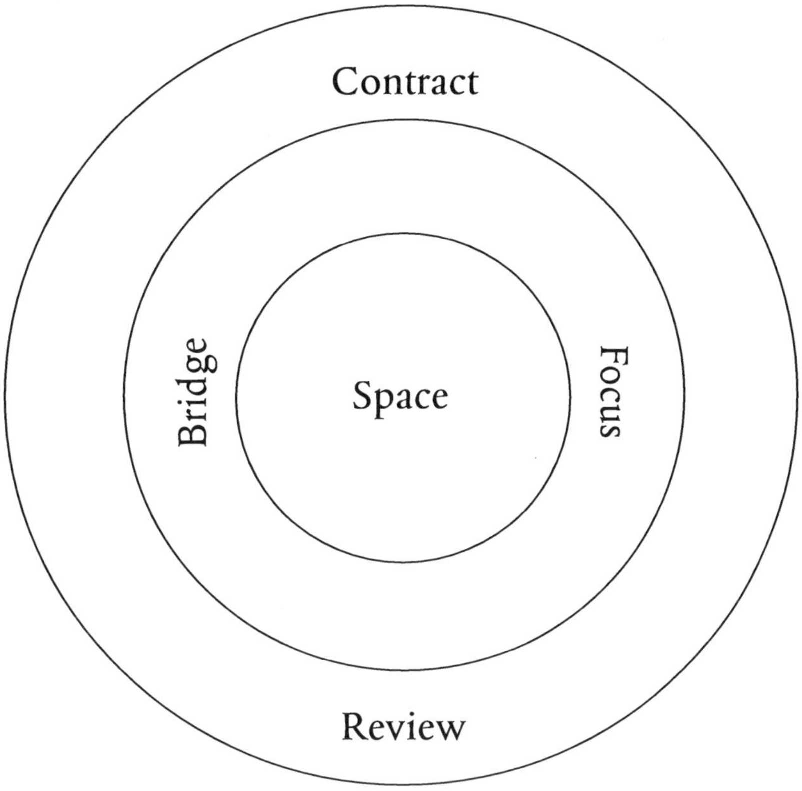

Figure 1.2: The cyclical model as a container. Copyright Steve Page and Val Wosket (2001)

> For example I [Steve] quite commonly invite supervisees to speak the unspeakable – say what they sometimes think but would, quite rightly, never say to their client. I encourage them to exaggerate, to be outrageous if they wish. This can be fun, but has a deadly serious purpose. It often liberates the counsellor who is stuck in some way. However I need to be clear that the supervisee and I both understand that this is in no way an encouragement to speak in this way to the client. The clear and explicit boundary between time for exploration and time for application helps me to feel confident that this distinction is understood. It also seems to help supervisees to feel able to be more playful. Playfulness, fun, inventiveness all fertilise the ground in which the seeds of creativity lie.

When we come to the 'bridge' then the very act of attending to the process of application tends to require a rational thinking mode. This imposes what is a healthy form of discipline upon supervisor and supervisee together. It acts as a reminder that ultimately we are there in the service of the client. If we are not able to make the shift into this way of thinking this suggests that something has not been fully attended to or resolved within the 'space'. Thus it acts as a kind of chaos detection device.

The other stage that is in the second layer out from the centre in the container version of the model is 'focus', where the supervisee, if necessary with assistance from the supervisor but often on their own, identifies that to which attention will be given. Since we first created this model we have enjoyed playing with 'focus' and also observing how different supervisees use this part of the process. Some practitioners arrive having prepared diligently, outlining what they want to focus on, what their priorities are and as they move from one focus to the next make clear what they want from supervision. Others are somewhat looser, but nevertheless with an idea of what they want and where the attention needs to be given.

> This brings to mind an example of supervision chaos with an experienced counsellor (whom I shall call 'Jack') in the early stages of our supervision relationship. As we started supervision I found myself feeling increasingly bewildered and struggling to get hold of anything tangible in our discussions. I couldn't get a sense of the client in any meaningful way – I felt shut out, and somewhat mesmerised. This troubled me and I tried to raise it with Jack, but that didn't help – I think he simply felt hurt and misunderstood. He was bringing client work and talking about it but I felt that we were not engaged in a useful supervision process. I went back to the original version of our model and realised that I had no sense of focus, so introduced that notion. The next session Jack provided a much clearer focus, but the same thing happened – after 30 minutes I felt bewildered, I didn't know what to do and I felt that my interventions were becoming exasperated and somewhat critical and punitive in tone.
>
> I recall raising the possibility of deciding that the relationship simply wasn't working and stopping, but neither of us wanted that. It transpired that Jack had sought me out because of my reputation for clarity – and was still hopeful! I was basically too obstinate to give up – when faced with a challenge I want to find a way through. In supervision of my supervision we returned to the model and, amongst other things, looked at the different sub-components of 'focus'. Out of this emerged the idea of asking Jack to bring in an audiotape of a session. Now this may all sound very simple but I want to remind you that in this supervision relationship the fog was thick for all involved. In this circumstance any glimmering of light is very welcome. There then followed a lengthy period of trust building in the relationship while the audio tapes of counselling sessions provided a tangible way of starting to explore what was going on within the counselling sessions in a way with which I felt comfortable.

> Again my chaos detector was at work. I could have tried to tackle this difficulty as supervisee transference, a counter-productive defensive strategy, a difficulty in our relationship dynamics or an indicator of reason for concern about his practice. Given the resulting progress I am pleased that my supervisor and I instinctively took a primarily task-oriented approach. Once the work was better established it was possible for Jack and I to look back and acknowledge some of the aspects of each of us, and the differences between us, that had contributed to those early difficulties. I think of it as an example of the 'focus' acting as the container of something that was interfering with effective supervision – chaos if you will.

The outer circle of the container version of the model contains two elements: 'contract' and 'review'. Once the initial contract has been agreed these two become part of what is often a seamless process of review and re-contracting. From a containment perspective they provide the functional working agreement between two adult practitioners. If used explicitly this creates a shared understanding of what will take place. If any element of chaos enters this at all, if what is agreed does not take place, or it does not achieve what is intended, this should be readily apparent and can be addressed.

In summary, in thinking about our model in this particular way it becomes apparent that there is great capacity for uncertainty, spontaneity, and many dimensions in what occurs at the centre, in the 'space'. However, this is dependent upon and in contrast to a need for increasing clarity as we move out into 'focus' and 'bridge' and then more clarity still as we come to 'contract' and 'review'.

Finally we will draw some conclusions from this discussion. Perhaps, as Crouch (1997) has implied, the true test of any model or theory is whether it provides an affirmative response to the following question: 'can I make it come alive, can I make it a part of my personal, and then my practitioner "bones"?' (p.ix). Supervisors who have an eye too firmly fixed on the mechanics of a model may miss paying sufficient attention to that which humanises it, that is, the relationship. A model is only a small part of what competent supervisors offer to their supervisees. A model provides a framework and a map for the supervisory tasks and process. The quality of the work that takes place within that framework is largely governed by other, less tangible, things. In particular, models are technical procedures that require to be humanised in order to work effectively and to be palatable to the recipient. In the process of being humanised a model of supervision should cease to be a close reflection of a particular school, originator or theoretical doctrine and instead become a vehicle through which the individual practitioner finds expression for their own unique abilities and qualities as a supervisor.

The cyclical model of counsellor supervision attempts to deal with this tension by providing a balance between a structure that is clear and well defined and a process that is flexible and adaptable. It can be used in a minimalist way as a loose framework for organising the supervision process or as a highly structured and detailed exposition of the tasks and functions of supervision with precise interventions for each of its 5 stages and 25 sub-steps. Thus for trainee supervisors it is intended to provide safety, containment and direction together with a repertoire of interventions sufficient to answer that question which is likely to trouble any of us at some stage of the learning process: 'What do I do *now*?' As students of supervision advance and develop their own individual strengths and styles of working, the model becomes one that encourages freedom and offers room for experimentation rather than one that limits and constrains.

A good working model, as defined by Egan (1984), is 'a framework or cognitive map with "delivery" potential' (p.25). The most effective supervision models are those that set supervisors free, rather than imprison them. An effective supervision model should provide just enough in the way of structure and guidance to enable the supervisor to tolerate and work with the unknown and unexpected in supervisees and their clients. An effective model is one that can be tailored to the supervisor's unique style and character so that it is worn as a close-fitting glove that takes on the shape and form of the hand within it, rather than forcing the hand into a crooked or unnatural form.

Over-reliance on a supervision model may diminish or even obliterate much of what the supervisor has already available within his or her natural helping repertoire. Supervisors should therefore be prepared to abandon their supervision models when original and creative responses to supervisees are called for. Because much of the territory of supervision concerns exploring the unknown this requires risk taking by both supervisor and supervisee. A key task for the supervisor is to help the counsellor develop the courage and willingness to face the unknown in themselves and their clients. In so doing, the supervisor will, at times, also need to face the unknown in themselves. In particular, the effective supervisor needs to risk appearing foolish and vulnerable for out of vulnerability and fallibility come creativity and movement. This is as true of supervision as it is of counselling. At times, in supervision, as in counselling, the most powerful interventions are those which emanate from unfiltered compassion and humanity extended from one unique human being to another (Wosket 1999). As Hycner (1991) has asserted 'openness to genuine meeting always means a willingness to encounter the unexpected, the existential unknown between persons, and leaving the security of one's method and theory' (p.22).

> Once, and only once in eight years, my supervisor cried with me as I [Val] wept in despair and frustration over my client who was so determined to end her own life. My supervisor was as surprised as I was by her tears and exclaimed 'I don't know what suddenly hit me there.' But for me, in witnessing her tears I learned that I could touch my supervisor deeply in an unguarded moment. And this being so,

might it not also become possible that I could, perhaps, reach that very far away place in my client where compassion could take a hold and maybe, just maybe, make a difference? This gave me the courage to continue and to carry some hope for my client when she had none for herself. Unwittingly, and out of her own vulnerability, my supervisor had provided the perfect response to my difficulty.

Endnote

1 For anyone not familiar with this model it has five basic stages, each of which has five sub-units. The basic stages are: contract – the formal agreement between supervisor and supervisee; focus – the identified issue or client material which is to be explored; space – the opportunity to explore the material in a reflective manner; bridge – the link between the discussion in 'space' and the next contact with the client; review – the review of the work, supervisory relationship and contract. For a full description refer to Page and Wosket (2001).

References

Bly, R. (1988) *A Little Book on the Human Shadow.* (Edited by William Booth.) San Francisco, CA: Harper and Row.

Borders, L. D. (1992) 'Learning to think like a supervisor.' *The Clinical Supervisor 10,* 2, 135–148.

Carr, J. T. (1994) 'Three cases.' In E. Messner, J. E. Groves and J. H. Schwartz (eds) *What Therapists Learn about Themselves and How they Learn it: Autognosis.* Northvale, NJ: Jason Aronson.

Connor, M. (1994) *Training the Counsellor: An Integrative Model.* London: Routledge.

Corey, G., Corey, M. S. and Callanan, P. (1993) *Issues and Ethics in the Helping Professions* (fourth edition). California: Brooks/Cole.

Crouch, A. (1997) *Inside Counselling: Becoming and Being a Professional Counsellor.* London: Sage.

Dryden, W., Horton, I. and Mearns, D. (1995) *Issues in Professional Counsellor Training.* London: Cassell.

Egan, G. (1984) 'People in systems: a comprehensive model of psychosocial education and training.' In D. Larson (ed) *Teaching Psychological Skills: Models for Giving Psychology Away.* Monterey: Brooks/Cole.

Feltham, C. (1995) *What is Counselling?* London: Sage.

Feltham, C. (1996) 'Beyond denial, myth and superstition in the counselling professions.' In R. Bayne, I. Horton and J. Bimrose (eds) *New Directions in Counselling.* London: Routledge.

Feltham, C. (1997) 'Challenging the core theoretical model.' *Counselling 8,* 2, 121–125.

Feltham, C. (1999) (ed) *Controversies in Psychotherapy and Counselling.* London: Sage.

Feltham, C. (2000) 'Counselling supervision: baselines, problems and possibilities.' In B. Lawton and C. Feltham (eds) *Taking Supervision Forward: Enquiries and Trends in Counselling and Psychotherapy.* London: Sage.

Frank, J. D. (1989) 'Non-specific aspects of treatment: the view of a psychotherapist.' In M. Shepherd and N. Sartorius (eds) *Non-Specific Aspects of Treatment.* Toronto: Hans Huber.

Goldfried, M. R. and Pradawer, W. (1982) 'Current status and future directions in psychotherapy.' In M. R. Goldfried (ed) *Converging Themes in Psychotherapy: Trends in Psychodynamic, Humanistic and Behavioral Practice.* New York: Springer.

Hawkins, P. and Shohet, R. (1989) *Supervision in the Helping Professions.* Milton Keynes: Open University Press.

Hobson, R. F. (1985) *Forms of Feeling: The Heart of Psychotherapy.* London: Routledge.

Horton, I. (1996) 'Towards the construction of a model of counselling.' In R. Bayne, I. Horton and J. Bimrose (eds) *New Directions in Counselling.* London: Routledge.

Hycner, R. H. (1991) *Between Person and Person: Towards a Dialogical Psychotherapy.* Highland, NY: The Gestalt Journal.

Johnson, R. A. (1991) *Owning Your Own Shadow: Understanding the Dark Side of the Psyche.* San Francisco, CA: Harper Collins.

Jung, C. G. (1959) *Aion.* (Collected works volume 9, part II.) London: Routledge and Kegan Paul.

Kaslow, F. W. (1986) 'Supervision, consultation and staff training – creative teaching/learning processes in the mental health profession.' In F. W. Kaslow (ed) *Supervision and Training Models, Dilemmas and Challenges.* Binghamton, NY: Haworth Press.

Lewin, R. A. (1996) *Compassion: The Core Value that Animates Psychotherapy.* Northvale, NJ: Jason Aronson.

O'Connell, B. and Jones, C. (1997) 'Solution focused supervision.' *Counselling 8,* 4, 289–292.

Page, S. (1999a) *The Shadow and the Counsellor: Working with Darker Aspects of the Person, Role and Profession.* London: Routledge.

Page, S. (1999b) *Qualitative Study of the Experiences of Members of a Supervision Group based upon the Cyclical Model of Counsellor Supervision.* An unpublished work in progress summary, presented as poster at British Association for Counselling Research Conference 1999. Copies available from Steve Page, University of Hull, Hull, HU6 7RX, UK.

Page, S. and Wosket, V. (1994) *Supervising the Counsellor: A Cyclical Model.* London: Routledge.

Page, S. and Wosket, V. (2001) *Supervising the Counsellor: A Cyclical Model* (second edition) London: Routledge.

Selekman, M. and Todd, T. (1995) 'Co-creating a context for change in the supervisory system: the solution focused supervision model.' *Journal of Systemic Therapies 14,* 3, 21–33.

Skovholt, T. M. and Rønnestad, M. H. (1995) *The Evolving Professional Self: Stages and Themes in Therapist and Counselor Development.* Chichester: Wiley.

Wheeler, S. (1998) 'Challenging the core theoretical model: a reply to Colin Feltham.' *Counselling 9*, 2, 134–138.

Wilkins, P. (1997) *Personal and Professional Development for Counsellors.* London: Sage.

Wosket, V. (1999) *The Therapeutic Use of Self: Counselling Practice, Research and Supervision.* London: Routledge.

Wosket, V. (2000) 'Integration and eclecticism in supervision.' In S. Palmer and R. Woolfe (eds) *Integrative and Eclectic Counselling and Psychotherapy.* London: Sage.

Chapter 2

Narrative Approaches to Supervision

Jane Speedy

Introduction

There has been a recent 'narrative turn of the globe' of such significance that it has caused the psychologist, Jerome Bruner (1986), to wonder whether human beings might be better described as 'homo fabulans' than 'homo sapiens'. I am very attracted by this narrative turn and its impact on counselling practice, research and theory. I have always loved stories. I have always lived a 'storied' life and been a respectful, creative and curious audience for the stories my clients – trainees and supervisees – have shared with me. In another life, or perhaps later on in this one, I might have been a storyteller, a 'cantadora' like Clarrisa Pinkola Estes (1993), who tells us:

> Among my people, questions are often answered with stories. The first story almost always evokes another, which summons another, until the answer to the question has become several stories long. A sequence of tales is thought to offer broader and deeper insight than a single story alone. (p.1)

I have become particularly interested in the influence that narrative approaches might have on counselling supervision. I am a supervisor myself and also a trainer of supervisees and supervisors. I am convinced that supervision is a professional arena that is enriched by narrative ways of knowing, understanding and 'positioning' ourselves. It is not really possible to provide anything more than a brief introduction to the narrative therapies here. If these ideas capture your imagination, there is a growing literature in this field (see Freedman and Combs 1996; McLeod 1997; Monk *et al.* 1997; White and Epston 1991). Perhaps it might help if I started by 'positioning' myself and outlining some of the tenets and metaphors of a socially constructed, storied world. I might then make some suggestions about their relevance to counselling supervision.

Living in a storied world

There are various ways of understanding and describing the narrative therapies and their origins. John McLeod gives a very good summary of all this in the second edition of *An Introduction to Counselling* (McLeod 1998). There is often confusion between the words 'narrative' and 'story'. For my purposes, I shall use 'narrative' as an overarching term and the word 'story' for the many tales we tell and re-tell about our endeavours and ourselves. Having limited space, I will take up a 'social constructivist' position as I tell the story of counselling, although there are other versions of this story.

Counselling was developed within the post-war western culture of individualism and positivism; a 'modern' era in which people were attempting to establish certainties about the nature of the world and of human beings, their potentials and their everyday behaviours. Alongside the 'grand narratives' of humanism, behaviourism, and so on, some social theorists and counselling practitioners were also emerging whose understanding of what it meant to be a person was more fluid. They viewed counselling and psychotherapy, alongside other human endeavours, as culturally and socially, as well as individually and psychologically, constructed phenomena (see McLeod 1997; McNamee and Gergen 1992). Their image of being and becoming a person was culturally embedded. People were defined, liberated and limited by their own 'moral visions' (Christopher 1996). Personal change was made possible not by finding their 'true' or authentic selves, but by developing a sense of agency and by reconstructing or reinventing themselves and their endeavours within the parameters of their culture.

These 'post-modernists', as we might choose to call them, abandoned the certainties of 'grand narratives', perceiving them only as culturally or temporally dominant versions amongst a diversity of narratives, local knowledge and possible stories. To quote Gergen: 'The postmodern argument is not against the various schools of therapy, only against their posture of authoritative truth.' (McNamee and Gergen 1992, p.57.)

Post-modernists and social constructivists are sometimes accused of relativism or nihilism. This does not seem a very accurate account of the ways these ideas have influenced counselling and psychotherapy. Feminist and narrative therapists have valued everyday stories and hidden voices (what we might call narrative knowing) as much as abstract constructs, theoretical models and dominant voices (sometimes called paradigmatic knowing). They have given equal emphasis to hidden, as well as to dominant voices.

Clients, counsellors, supervisees and supervisors can only be understood within their context, to which they bring not only themselves, but also what Geertz (1983) describes as their 'webs of significance'. People are no longer seen as unique individuals at the centre of their systems (see Egan and Cowan 1979 for a very 'individualistic' and western representation of 'people in systems') but rather as unique, fluid individuals amidst a constantly changing web of connections and stories. It is as if this interconnectedness and interweaving of stories moves the moral stance of the counselling, or indeed, the supervisory relationship out of the therapy room and into the global community. The context, history and culture of the supervisor, supervisee and client are inescapably, rather than potentially, available in supervision. The emphasis on 'globalisation' that characterises the narrative therapies strongly counters the rather individualistic 'bystander syndrome' (Clarkson 1996) of which more traditional approaches to counselling and psychotherapy have sometimes been accused.

The story of the narrative therapists working in New Zealand is a prime example of the value of 'narrative knowing'. These therapists set out to 'deconstruct' western versions of individual potential and 'reconstruct' more collectively based stories about who we are. These resonated with the stories that Maori peoples told about themselves. Many of the exercises that I now use to introduce narrative approaches to supervision have come from Australia and New Zealand. (See Monk *et al.* 1997; White and Epston 1991.)

'Positioning ourselves'

The vocabulary of 'narrative knowing' is common across the academic traditions of anthropology, linguistics, philosophy, psychology and literary theory, but may be unfamiliar to many counsellors. It is worth spending a bit of time 'deconstructing' this terminology.

Narrative therapists are interested in exploring how people are 'positioned' in relation to dominant or local narratives (how their stories interweave and are different from or influenced by socially and culturally significant versions). Therapists listen curiously (adopting a spirit of naïve inquiry, a not-knowing stance) to the positions people assume and explore the history of these positions. They invite people to adopt a respectful curiosity about their own stories and about how their stories change in different contexts, or over time. They acknowledge and make explicit the way stories change in the space between therapist and client. In this way stories and 'truths' are continually being 'co-created' between people.

They engage their clients in 'deconstructing conversations' (exploring meanings, possible inconsistencies, assumptions and histories). They ask 'externalising questions' that separate the narrator from the story (the story, or problem becomes an 'it' that client and therapist can explore together). This allows the narrator (the client or supervisee) to separate himself or herself from the problem or 'character' in the story and see 'it' from a range of different positions. It may be that unique outcomes (situations where the story can be different, or different ways of constructing the same story) are uncovered in this process. The narrator can consider situating themselves differently and experiment with the possibility of retelling or re-authoring the story.

Here is a short, concrete example from my experience of supervising a supervisor:

> *Curious listener*: So how do you 'position' yourself as a supervisor? [Listening curiously and explicitly using narrative language.]
>
> *Speaker*: I like to think of myself as something of a rebel.
>
> *Curious listener*: Is that a new position or has it been around a while?
>
> *Speaker*: Oh, it's old, old stuff, left over from my school days.
>
> *Curious listener*: So, it's left over, but nonetheless 'rebel' is a position that you like to think of yourself in. Has it been a useful position? [Externalising 'rebel' into a position rather than an innate characteristic and deconstructing the history of 'rebel'.]
>
> *Speaker*: Well it means I don't have to belong to any particular 'group think' or be swept along by the latest trend. Only a fainthearted rebel, mind you, but it's served me well. Well most of the time.
>
> *Curious listener*: Most of the time. Can you tell me some of the ways this 'fainthearted rebel' might have got in the way? [Deconstructing rebel and looking for outcomes.]
>
> *Speaker*: Well, it's the place where I nearly always start, in professional settings, and sometimes I don't need to ... sometimes I lose the plot.
>
> *Curious listener*: So it's your starting position in professional settings, but perhaps not in other settings?
>
> *Speaker*: Good god, I'm a wimp at home!

This is only a short extract, but perhaps serves to illustrate some of the ways that narrative terms can be specifically used and shared, that issues can be placed in their 'history' and context and can be externalised by both listener and speaker. This dialogue went on to examine the value of faintheartedness, a great strength for this particular supervisor.

So, if we were to 'reconstruct' the stories we tell ourselves about counselling supervision, what might that look like and how might that help our clients and us?

Positioning counselling supervision

The proliferation of schools, tribes and territories within counselling seems to be spilling over to the supervisory context. There seem to be several new approaches or 'supervision designer labels' being offered and I have no desire to add another one. I am offering a narrative approach as a way of positioning ourselves as supervisors and as a means of developing a different 'take' on what we already do. I will be introducing some activities to illustrate this way of working, but I am not really offering tricks or techniques to add to your repertoire. I am suggesting that a narrative world view, a sense of the world as a storied place to live and work, provides a different position from which to explore the very human endeavours of counselling, psychotherapy and supervision. I have no intention, for the moment, of abandoning the models I have found useful in developing my 'helicopter skills' as a counselling supervisor, whether these are developmental, process, cyclical or functional stories about what I do. I am also aware that these are only stories and that they may be reinvented, recreated or jettisoned altogether in light of new contexts or understandings.

In my own everyday practice as a supervisor, Hawkins and Shohet's six- (or seven-) eyed 'process' model (1989) and Inskipp and Proctor's (1993; 1995) functional model (to which Hazel Johns has added a 'creative' function (1996)) are the checklists I carry with me most often in my 'supervisor's toolkit'. I have found the story metaphor a helpful integrating tool when working with supervisors who uphold different, seemingly oppositional, professional beliefs and values. My learning from facilitating groups of experienced supervisors undertaking the MSc in counselling supervision and training at the University of Bristol has been that listening curiously to each other about our professional stories has enabled us to work together more effectively. Here is an experiential exercise we use.

Activity One: Deconstructing our 'supervision stories'

The listener adopts a stance of persistent and genuine curiosity and invites the speaker to offer the preferred description of him or herself as supervisors. The listener helps the speaker to uncover the history and development of this description during the course of the speaker's professional life. To make the thinking behind this activity explicit, I think it is a useful way of highlighting that our professional allegiances, so often hard won and hard fought, are temporally, historically and culturally embedded. They are also restricted by our world view, as physicist Stephen Hawking (1988) adroitly reminds us, with the observation that we remember our pasts more readily than our futures! The language of 'preferred' description also invites possibility, opportunity, change and a multiplicity of co-existing stories.

Some useful openers and questions:

- I am really curious about... (for example, what 'feminist' might mean to you).
- I'd like to know more about... (how 'feminism' informs supervision).
- How is this description currently useful in...? (for example, supervising male therapists).
- In what ways does this description work for you now in...? (for example, your particular agency).
- What effect has this conversation had on your preferred description? (for example, is 'feminism' qualified or clarified in any way?).
- How might you prefer to describe yourself in ten years time? (that is, keeping possibility and change on the agenda).

It seems that in deconstructing and co-creating the stories we tell ourselves and each other about counselling supervision, a number of shifts in understanding are able to take place. People gain insights into the assumptions and influences behind their stories and often make quite substantial changes to their preferred descriptions. People deconstruct their 'local knowledges' about counselling supervision and explore 'sacred cows' such as core theoretical models, parallel processes and developmental stages more critically and more curiously. Most significantly, people from a range of counselling tribes and territories seem to respond well to the story metaphor and develop a curiosity about mutualities, differences, contexts and 'cultural embededness' rather than dig themselves into entrenched or conflicting positions.

Language and positioning in counselling supervision

From a post-modernist standpoint the language we use not only describes, but also determines our world. Introducing explicitly narrative terminology changes the way we are 'situated' within counselling supervision. We have barely begun to explore the differences that reconstructing ourselves as critical audience (supervisor) and narrator (supervisee) make to the supervisory relationship. Situating ourselves within the discourse of storymaking seems to alter the positions that are available to us.

Recognising the counsellor/client relationship as a 'narrated relationship' recreated in the re-telling offers a number of possibilities and legitimacies. The story metaphor clarifies the 'make-believe' nature of the supervisor's relationship with the client. Grandiose tendencies on the part of supervisors to make up heroic stories inside their own heads about the successful outcomes for the client 'if only they had had me as their counsellor' can be acknowledged and countered, rather than ignored or condemned, within this discourse of make-believe.

The supervisor's position as 'audience' and 'curious listener' also makes an impact on supervisory relationships. Regardless of the number of props, videos and accompanying notes that they may have as aids to their authenticity, the role of the narrator is to re-tell the story to suit the cultural context. This will always be a subjective account. The audience can only listen, but in so doing, they are also co-creating the story, countering the story and wondering about other possible stories the narrator might have told. In most, but not all theatrical settings, the audience do not participate in the performance but are nonetheless an integral part of it. They not only provide feedback about the story unfolding onstage, they can also make or break a production – a powerful metaphor indeed!

Assuming these positions seems to provide a different landscape in a number of ways. The story metaphor enhances and legitimates our sense of supervision as creative playspace. It also seems to strengthen our sense of moral commitment to and connectedness with the client whose story is being told. (See Wheeler and King (1999) for a disquieting glance at our current sense of responsibility in counselling supervision.) It is as if, paradoxically, the ethical purposes and responsibilities of counselling supervisors and supervisees are heightened by an increased awareness that 'it is only a story', one of an infinite number of possible, interconnecting stories.

The moral philosopher, Jonathan Glover, is convinced that our day-to-day ethics and codes of practice ought to be informed by the extraordinary stories of atrocities and disasters and of the ways that human nature can go wrong:

> For many of us catastrophes are remote from everyday life. Luckily, the ethics of preventing atrocities are extensions of the ethics of everyday life. At the supermarket people do not park in the disabled space because they do not want a disabled person to have the indignity and difficulty of struggling to carry groceries. They may also not want to be somebody who is mean enough to cause this. The moral resources here are the same as those needed in moral emergencies. (Glover 1999, p.408.)

In expanding our moral imaginations and in being mindful of our everyday professional responsibilities, supervisors and supervisees alike may be better placed for dealing with 'moral emergencies'.

Activity Two: 'Storied' supervision

A second experiential exercise allows the supervisor to position themselves as 'critical audience' to the narrator of the supervision story and listen curiously. The supervisor explicitly uses 'storied language' and invites curiosity and potential re-authoring from the supervisee or narrator.

Some useful suggestions and questions:

- Does this story have a title?
- What are the names of the central characters in the story?
- If your client were telling this story what would the title be?
- If you were a character in your client's story, who would you be?

Or, in a more 'six-eyed' frame: You're telling me a lot of stories ... There's the client and his issue / your issue with the client /you, your organisation, its issues and me ... Which story do you want to focus on for the moment?

- Are those the positions you usually take when you tell supervision stories?
- If I went now and told this story to my supervisor, what do you imagine I might say?

People are frequently surprised by this way of working. It feels quite playful and creative; yet working more lightly does not mean the same as working less mindfully. It is hard for some of us to move out of our traditional worldviews and accept that a 'narrative way of knowing' might involve a great deal of not knowing how other people construct their worlds. The supervisor will be listening curiously and may help the narrator to uncover inconsistencies or unique outcomes. It may be hard for experienced practitioners to accept that sometimes all we have to offer as supervisors is a spirit of naïve inquiry and a sense of possibility in the way we position ourselves in the telling and re-telling of our stories.

An aspect of this work that people find strange (when I demonstrate it before an audience) is the amount of questioning. Although my questions are 'warm, respectful and "quite person-centred"' they certainly keep coming! It is, indeed, a very inquisitive, although, I hope, not inquisitorial way of working. All the deconstructing of meanings and positions takes place explicitly in the space between supervisor and supervisee. I suspect it seemed person-centred in my case because that is the therapeutic tradition from which I come. A narrative approach under different management, as it were, might equally and legitimately take on a Jungian or Kohutian appearance.

Endnote

This chapter represents a taste of some 'work in progress' rather than a neatly packaged final product. It is not my intention ever to produce a full-blown, brand-named, copper-bottomed, trademarked narrative core theoretical model of supervision (although the irony and paradox of such a story is not entirely lost on me!). My own world-view has, nonetheless, been changed irretrievably as I have come into contact with narrative ideas, as has my understanding about the work that we do and the stories we tell ourselves as counsellors, supervisors and trainers. My experience and understanding of the potency and influence of narrative approaches within counselling, counselling supervision, counselling training and counselling research continues to expand and develop all the time. I should also like to take this opportunity to thank my colleagues at the University of Bristol for their contributions to this 'work in progress'.

References

Bruner, J. (1986) *Actual Minds, Possible Worlds.* Cambridge, MA: Harvard University Press.

Christopher, J. C. (1996) 'Counseling's inescapable moral visions.' *Journal of Counseling and Development 75*, 17–25.

Clarkson, P. (1996) *The Bystander (An End to Innocence in Human Relationships?).* London: Whurr.

Egan, G. and Cowan, M. (1979) *People in Systems: A Model for Development in the Human-service Professions and Education.* Pacific Grove, CA: Brooks Cole.

Freedman, J. and Combs, G. (1996) *Narrative Therapy: The Social Construction of Preferred Realities.* New York: Norton.

Geertz, C. (1983) *Local Knowledge: Further Essays in Interpretative Anthropology.* New York: Basic Books.

Gergen, K. (1992) 'The post-modern adventure.' *Family Therapy Networker 52*, 56–58.

Glover, J. (1999) *Humanity: A Moral History of the Twentieth Century.* London: Jonathan Cape.

Hawking, S. (1988) *A Brief History of Time: From the Big Bang to Black Holes.* London: Bantam.

Hawkins, P. and Shohet, R. (1989) *Supervision in the Helping Professions.* Milton Keynes: Open University Press.

Inskipp, F. and Proctor, B. (1993) *The Art, Craft and Tasks of Counselling Supervision. Part 1: Making the Most of Supervision.* Twickenham: Cascade.

Inskipp, F. and Proctor, B. (1995) *The Art, Craft and Tasks of Counselling Supervision. Part 2: Becoming A Supervisor.* Twickenham: Cascade.

Johns, H. (1996) *Personal Development in Councelling Training.* London: Cassell.

McLeod, J. (1997) *Narrative and Psychotherapy.* London: Sage.

McLeod, J. (1998) *An Introduction to Counselling.* (Second edition.) Buckingham: Open University Press.

McNamee, S. and Gergen, K. (1992) (eds) *Therapy as Social Construction.* London: Sage.

Monk, G., Winslade, J., Crocket, K. and Epston, D. (1997) (eds) *Narrative Therapy in Practice: The Archaeology of Hope.* San Francisco, CA: Jossey Bass.

Pinkola Estes, C. (1993) *The Gift of Story: A Wise Tale About What is Enough.* London: Rider.

Wheeler, S. and King, D. (1999) 'The responsibilities of counsellor supervisors: a qualitative study.' *British Journal of Guidance and Counselling 27*, 2, 215–231.

White, M. and Epston, D. (1991) *Narrative Means to Therapeutic End.* New York: Norton.

Chapter 3

A Collaborative Model of Supervision

Vanja Orlans and Dagmar Edwards

Introduction

A number of different factors have contributed to our developing interest in supervision. First, we have both had many years of varied experience as supervisees, both in the course of our clinical training and beyond. Some of these experiences were good ones – we felt deeply supported and challenged in our clinical work with the supervisory experiences making a major contribution to our professional development – while others left us with questions about the process as a whole. Also relevant are our many years of clinical experience with our clients, the development of our own skills as supervisors, both through training and through practice, the writing of a dissertation and some early 'pilot' research work designed to explore the process of supervision in terms of learning, relationship and outcomes.

The wider professional field has also had an influence on our thinking about supervision. A perusal of the professional literature, journal articles and advertisements in professional publications over the last few years indicates a sharp increase in the awareness of supervision and related issues. Until fairly recently a key assumption would seem to have been that a qualification in clinical work, coupled with sufficient experience, provided the training necessary to be a supervisor. Now, however, we are seeing an increasing interest in the accreditation and accountability of professionals generally in the clinical field, and supervision as a potential professional area of expertise has become a part of this. Of significance also is the greater litigious environment in which we now work, and the move by professional bodies, as well as the government, to control the 'quality' of professional services on offer. All of these factors have played their part in motivating us to begin writing about the process of supervising as well as fuelling our interest in the design of learning opportunities for current and potential supervisors. In this chapter we present an overview of our current thinking and the implications of our ideas for practice. Our main focus is on the supervision of counselling and psychotherapeutic practitioners, but our ideas are relevant also to the broader supervision field.

Our interest in supervision falls broadly into two main areas: *the supervisory relationship* and *the learning process* within the context of supervision. These will be the focus points of this chapter. We shall present arguments as to why these interests are relevant to the quality of service which is provided to clients and what the implications might be for the training of supervisory approaches and skills. The ideas presented also form the basis of a training programme for supervisors which we have recently designed and are offering early in 2001.

An overview of the model

Our model of supervision encompasses a number of important dimensions which we see as interrelating with each other (see Figure 3.1 below). In our conceptualisation, we present the ultimate focus or 'outcome' as being *the quality of service to the client.* We make the assumption that our colleagues will agree with us that this is a valid focus and ultimate goal of the supervision process. The question then arises as to what factors may be identified which serve to support the highest quality service possible. Our own view is that this service is dependent on the quality of the ongoing learning, development and skill building which takes place in the context of the supervisory relationship, whether in a one-to-one or group setting.

From this perspective, and drawing on the Gestalt concepts of 'figure' and 'ground', the learning relationship is 'figure', and the various functions and contextual factors within a given supervisory framework move into the 'ground'. In terms of the relationship issue itself, we have identified two particular dimensions that are key to the issue of quality: First, *the supervisory relationship*, and second, *a set of collaborative principles and behaviours* which operate within, and which support, this relationship, and which in turn support the quality of service to the client. In terms of an ongoing process, it is clear that the dimensions of relationship and collaborative principles interrelate over time within the supervision process as a whole.

The supervisory relationship

In a previous article (Orlans and Edwards 1997) we have drawn attention to the fact that the literature on supervision does not provide much useful detail on the nature and development of an appropriate supervisory relationship in terms of its promotion of relevant learning as well as of a high quality service to clients. Yet, within the context of therapeutic work with clients, it is the quality and form of the relationship which is generally regarded as underpinning the ultimate

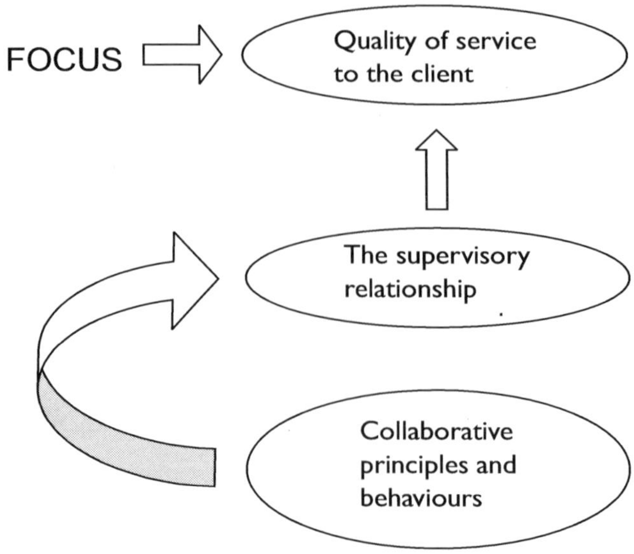

Figure 3.1: A collaborative model of supervision

effectiveness of the clinical process. It therefore seems slightly puzzling to us that relationship factors in supervision have not been more widely researched or written about – for example, we do not hear much about 'the supervisory alliance', or forms of 'transference' in supervision; at the same time, every clinical supervisor will be familiar with the notion of 'parallel process', recognising the ways in which the supervisory relationship takes on process dimensions of the original clinical work. A more radical perspective on this phenomenon is the idea that the clinical work might take on qualities of the supervision process. We shall return to this latter point in our later discussion.

Although several writers (Hawkins and Shohet 1989; Holloway 1995; Hunt 1986; Proctor 1994; Shohet and Wilmot 1991) make reference to the importance of the supervisory relationship, and outline in many instances some key aspects of the supervisory process between supervisor and supervisee, we feel that the relationship itself is never clearly presented as the overriding holding framework for potential learning and exploration. Holloway (1995), in her 'systems approach to supervision' presents seven dimensions of supervision, with 'the supervision relationship' highlighted as the central dimension, and referred to as the 'core factor'. She goes on to present a useful summary of research on relationship issues, in terms of the concepts of 'contract', 'phase', and 'structure', and also highlights the relevance of a 'reflection-in-action' approach as outlined by Donald Schön (1983). One is left, however, with the feeling that it is the supervisee who is the main focus, rather than 'the between', and with the feeling of an ongoing power imbalance in terms of the process. The model which we outline here is designed to contribute to an exploration and articulation of some significant relationship issues so that we can help supervisors to develop their skill base in a more systematic way.

Principles and behaviours of collaboration

The issue of 'collaboration' might be seen as a key integrating principle in terms of the developing supervisory relationship and the potential for learning that takes place within this relationship. We are talking here about the learning of *both* supervisee and supervisor, an issue which many professionals might view as self-evident, but which does not appear in an explicit way in the literature, and which is infrequently addressed in practice. Often, we get the feeling of an unbalanced approach in terms of learning requirements – the focus both in the literature as well as in practice seems more often to be on the learning of *the supervisee* than on that of the supervisor. Armed with a set of roles, responsibilities and skills, the supervisor sets out to attend to the learning of the supervisee – or so it seems to us that the story is told.

More interesting to us is the possibility and implication of a joint and explicit learning contract, both in terms of the underlying philosophy, and in terms of skill requirements. A truly joint venture with regard to learning within the supervisory relationship calls, in our view, for a transparency in the process, and for explicit attention to be paid to the developing relationship. This raises the question as to why we might want or need such a joint learning venture, and how this could possibly influence outcomes such as quality of service to the client. To answer this question, we turn to an examination of some of the key components of the learning process.

Reflections on the learning process

Psychological theory and research would suggest that learning is enhanced, and outcomes maximised, when the learner is involved in the process. This way the learner's motivation is engaged: they have an opportunity to co-create the structure of meaning inherent in the learning process, and are most likely to develop a commitment to achieving a set of learning goals. Also, this is an approach which, in the end, is likely to lead to better integration. As a whole, we are talking about a moving and ongoing process within a continuous spiral. We believe that this principle is generally accepted within education although its implementation may depend on the availability of certain resources such as time and teacher student ratio.

A further aspect of the learning process which is not generally given as much attention is the identification of different kinds of learning. Our interest here is specifically to do with the distinction between what has been termed 'single loop' and 'double loop', or 'Model I' and 'Model II' learning (Argyris 1970). The different forms of learning that human beings (and some animals) are capable of has been particularly well articulated by Gregory Bateson (1972). Bateson begins by outlining the properties of 'first order' and 'second order' change in the learning process, and the way in which human beings have the capacity to 'learn how to learn' – the 'second order' level. In documenting this ability, however, he also makes the point that, at this second order level, we act as though a broad range of problems can be solved by reference to certain assumptions and premises. While these in turn simplify the issue in that we now have fewer 'tasks' to deal with, they also cast us into a 'habitual' frame which, while useful in that it is an economical way to proceed, also constrains us in that we cease to question the core premises on which the original learning was based.

Bateson goes on to describe a further 'level' of learning, which he refers to as 'learning III', where the person becomes capable of freeing themselves from acquired habitual ways of functioning in the world. In this context, he quotes a Zen master as stating: 'To become accustomed to anything is a terrible thing' (p.304). Argyris and Schön's (1978) notion of 'double loop learning' approximates Bateson's idea of 'Level III'. Donald Schön in particular (1983) has developed some of this thinking and applied it to professional learning in a way which we find especially challenging for professionals working in the therapeutic setting, whether as counsellors, psychotherapists or supervisors.

Let us return then to the supervisory relationship and locate some of the ideas outlined above within that particular context. We would hold that the potential for 'double loop learning' should be held open in the supervisory relationship, both as a way of maximising learning within that setting, but also as a way of modelling possibilities for the work with clients. When clients come to see us it is usually the case that they are 'stuck' within certain patterns in their lives. If therapy or counselling works well they will have had to engage in some double loop learning along the way in order to liberate themselves from old premises and assumptions about their world. If we accept this process as valid in the therapeutic relationship, then we would argue that the same process needs to be mirrored in the supervisory relationship. At the same time, the nature of the supervisory relationship, with its attendant social roles and ethical/professional domains which have evolved over time, poses a particular challenge.

To truly *collaborate* on a joint learning venture could be experienced as risky for participants – at the very least it is likely to be filled with uncertainty for both supervisor and supervisee. It requires that the habitual maps which the person's present have so far evolved are laid open for perusal and further potential involvement in what might be experienced as a discontinuous direction – that is, new assumptions may need to be taken on and worked with. This process is, in our experience, both potentially very exciting, and also potentially uncomfortable. It is the kind of learning, however, that ensures freshness and openness to new experience and changed awareness, rather than sitting with what we already know and with what is often much more comfortable.

To summarise then, we are proposing a model of supervision which challenges supervisors to emerge from fixed roles and responsibilities in a way which makes us fully available for a relationship characterised by transparency and by the principles of collaboration and a commitment to 'Level III' learning (see Figure 3.2). According to Donald Schön's formulation, this requires of us a willingness to move beyond our 'technical rationality' – that is, beyond being passive receivers of knowledge and skill, and towards becoming active in the development of our own creativity. To work in this way requires of the supervisor a willingness to move out from behind a potentially more comfortable professional façade, towards a 'reflection-in-action' mode of being, where responsibility and accountability are more equally shared.

Having focused on the key principles of collaboration and learning, and some of the implications of these for the practice of supervision, we turn now to a review of some key skills, attitudes or behaviours which convert the principles described into potentially useful actions. We list some of these in Figure 3.2 below. Space precludes a detailed examination of each of these; in broad terms we are talking about a phenomenological attitude, where both supervisor and supervisee are willing to bracket their prejudices, attend to the description of what is available to the senses in the present moment, name 'unsaids' as well as other factors which

Collaboration as a key integrating principle

↕

Learning principles
Key focus on 'level III' learning

↕

Attitudes, behaviours, skills
Non-judgemental stance
Holistic presence
Descriptive phenomenology
Attention to power and transferential/countertransferential issues
Naming of difficult emotions (for example, anxiety)
Willingness to name relevant factors present in 'the field'

Figure 3.2: A collaborative model of supervision: principles, attitudes, behaviours and skills

might have a bearing on the relationship and on the work of supervision, and attend to the ebb and flow of energy as the process unfolds. In workshop settings, we use the immediacy of live practice experience, together with a number of exercises, to bring some of these issues to life. One particular exercise, and the rationale behind it, is described in the following section, and we invite the reader to try this exercise out for themselves.

The issue of 'size' in the supervisory relationship

In thinking about the evolvement of the supervisory role within the therapeutic setting, and the many aspects of this which are reflected both in the literature as well as in our own experiences of the process, we have developed a number of exercises and approaches which attempt to illuminate some key issues in a lively and experiential way, and which also enable supervisors to become more courageous in holding relationship issues as 'figure' in the course of their work. One of these ideas involves focusing on 'size' within the supervisory relationship. In doing so we are taking a very 'literal' approach to a number of factors which can include power relations, felt age or regressed states, lack of confidence and anxiety, or the different experiential states of 'judging' or 'feeling judged'. Under each of these conditions, if we tune into our physical sensations, we will find that our experience of our own size will generally vary.

Under certain conditions, or with some supervisors, we might feel 'small', or if we do not respect the supervisor we might feel 'big'. Where we feel, as the supervisor, that we are responsible for the supervisee's clinical work and that we are 'in charge' of the ethics of the matter, then we might feel 'big'. If all this 'responsibility' sits like concrete on our shoulders, making us feel very anxious or (literally) 'worn down', then we would be more likely to feel 'small'. So, by utilising the dimension of 'size', it make it possible very rapidly to tune into a range of important issues, some of which are even likely to be outside of our conscious experience at the time. Through the development of our awareness in this way we can bring new aspects of experience into focus, make them transparent, and figure out how to deal with these in a creative way. Importantly, we can do this figuring out *overtly* in the context of the supervisory relationship.

In training settings, we might invite participants, first, to turn to the person next to them and muse silently on the issue of 'size' between them and the other person – to notice their own sensations, their feelings, any images which emerged. We might then invite people to discuss their experience with their partner. There is usually some very lively 'unpacking' of what that part of the exercise had thrown up – lots of noise and a high level of energy in the room! We then ask people to imagine themselves with a supervisee and muse on the issue of size in a similar way. Again, we make space for some sharing within each dyad.

From the feedback we get it seems that many people experience this exercise as extremely powerful. It raises a number of issues, both personal and more general. These include the perceived 'risk' involved in being willing to stand at the edge of our own vulnerability, with a willingness to have our own anxiety or personal struggles made more visible. At the broader level of analysis, there is often discussion, for example, of potential differences with supervisees at different levels of training. It has been suggested that with beginning therapists or counsellors, it might be more appropriate for the supervisor to be 'big' in the relationship. There is also the issue, however, of whether 'big' means 'more supportive', or whether this suggestion is a rationalisation of the supervisor's need to keep control under conditions of uncertainty.

We are not advocating any 'rights' or 'wrongs' in exploring these issues – rather, we believe that it is important to open these up to our awareness in a more focused way, so that we can explore a range of processes and comment on their potential effectiveness. Using this kind of approach, we expand our range of intervention possibilities and open the way for experiments in our practice which can bring freshness and new insights to our work.

References

Argyris, C. (1970) *Intervention Theory and Method: A Behavioral Science View*. Reading, MA: Addison-Wesley.

Argyris, C. and Schön, D. A. (1978) *Theory in Practice: Increasing Professional Effectiveness.* San Francisco, CA: Jossey-Bass.

Bateson, G. (1972) *Steps to an Ecology of Mind.* New York: Ballantine Books.

Hawkins, P. and Shohet, R. (1989) *Supervision in the Helping Professions.* Milton Keynes: Open University Press.

Holloway, E. (1995) *Clinical Supervision: A Systems Approach.* Thousand Oaks, CA: Sage.

Hunt, P. (1986) *Supervision. Marriage Guidance.* Spring, 15–22.

Orlans, V. and Edwards, D. (1997) 'Focus and process in supervision.' *British Journal of Guidance and Counselling 25*, 409–415.

Proctor, B. (1994) 'Supervision – competence, confidence, accountability.' *British Journal of Guidance and Counselling 22*, 309–318.

Schön, D. A. (1983) *The Reflective Practitioner: How Professionals Think in Action.* London: Temple Smith.

Shohet, R. and Wilmot, J. (1991) 'The key issue in the supervision of counsellors: the supervisory relationship.' In W. Dryden and B. Thorne (eds) *Training and Supervision for Counselling in Action.* London: Sage.

Chapter 4

Supervision in and for Organisations

Michael Carroll

Introduction

Over the past five years I have moved from working directly with individuals as a counsellor and supervisor to working more directly with organisations. It has not been an easy transition and has involved me in changing individual frameworks, mindsets and theories to organisational ones. I was trained as a counsellor and supervisor and thought and worked within individual dynamics and paradigms. Not that I ignored the context from which the individual emerged, but it was not the primary focus of my work and therefore my way of assessing, intervening with and helping was through an individual lens. Much of that has changed since I began working for, in and with organisations. This chapter will summarise some of my recent thinking on how counselling, and supervision in particular, can be of help to contemporary organisations, institutions and companies in both private and public spheres.

Like individuals, organisations need supervision, badly. In many ways our organisations (whether educational, medical, business or religious) are much more in need of help than individuals. Counsellors and supervisors need to get more involved in organisations: it is so much easier to work with individuals, so much more comforting and comfortable, so positive to watch as they grow and develop. But we need to help our organisations too: in many ways they are more neglected than individuals are. Counsellors and supervisors have a unique contribution to make to modern organisations for two reasons. First, our British counselling and supervision training and practice is the best and most rounded I know. Were I advising someone to do his or her counselling or supervision training, I would recommend Britain as the place in which to study. I don't want to qualify that with any 'buts' and clearly I have no scientific evidence on which to base the above. Of course, there are 'buts' and lacunae in our counselling and supervision training and practice: however, I want that statement to stand on its own. Our counselling and supervision training and practice is the best there is. Second, our counsellors and supervisors are the best group of people, in my view, with their kitbag of philosophy, theory and strategies, to work within organisations today. I make no apology to clinical or occupational psychologists, or human resources or personnel: the best people to work with the people side of organisations today are counsellors and supervisors.

Management consultants, human resources and personnel practitioners and managers, all closely connected and involved with organisations, do not have the repertoire of skills, competencies, knowledge and experience of counsellors using supervision and variants of supervision. These supervision variants include sophisticated inventions such as executive coaching, mentoring, organisational development, outplacement and career counselling as well as team development and group work. Recently, I was asked to do a one-day training in 'group work' for consultants who were beginning to use groups in their learning methods. I suggested that training to work with groups demanded more than just a one-day training. Not at all, I was reminded, our consultants just need a few pointers and they will be fine. The expectation that a few simple learning strategies can qualify individuals to work in complex arenas is all too common in organisations.

Organisations desperately need people with the skills of counsellors and supervisors: there is no one else with this particular blend of knowledge and competencies. Organisations do not always know this or will let counsellors and supervisors close to them, but of all the professions I know counsellors/ supervisors (those who have those range of skills) are the best to work with contemporary organisations.

A fact from research (Berridge, Cooper and Highley-Marchington 1997) and a criticism of counselling (Pilgrim 1997) is that while counselling may make an individual different it has little impact on organisations. Introducing counselling in organisations, of itself, will not affect organisational change or culture or thinking. Can counsellors and supervisors begin to think of how they might work with, within and alongside organisations in order that they may be more human places in which to work and more healthy places where employees can develop and grow? The problem is summarised by Briskin (1998) in a book called *The Stirring of Soul in the Workplace*:

> To explore the challenge to the human soul in organisations is to build a bridge between the world of the personal, subjective and even unconscious elements of individual experience and the world of organisations that demand rationality, efficiency and personal sacrifice. (p.xii)

Getting close to organisations or their allowing supervisors into their sacred places is asking a lot.

Supervision and organisations

Seven reasons will be offered of how and why good supervisors could be of value in and to organisations today, summarised as follows:

1. To help organisations think through the theory behind what they do.
2. Questioning the myth that movement is always good.
3. Understanding the language of organisations.
4. Working with the emotional organisations (or the emotions within the organisation).
5. Remaining neutral (organisations as collusive places).
6. Focusing on what is good for the organisation.
7. Focusing on the individual within the organisation.

1. To help organisations think through the theory behind what they do

Theory rarely plays much of a part in the business of public and private organisations. Rarely do they ask what theory underlies a particular intervention or from what school does a consultant emerge, or what is the basis on which they should proceed or from what background a particular intervention comes. What works, or appears to work, is what matters. At a recent talk to HR Directors entitled 'Managing sensitive personnel issues in the workplace', a colleague upbraided me for not 'giving answers: that is what these people came for. You have given models and frameworks and theories but what they came here for are answers.' As if I, a total outsider to almost all their organisations, could provide ready-made, off-the-shelf, universal answers to complicated organisational issues. That is what is often expected: 'please give us the answers'.

Good supervisors know it is not about having the answers before the questions are asked. Consultants, managers and human resources, in some way that is not rational, still believe that answers are at the back of some book, or in some mind, somewhere. And, indeed, too many consultants emerge to meet the challenge and provide answers to questions asked, and indeed questions unasked. In doing so they make organisations dependent on them. As supervisor consultants we cannot take that route. Supervisors know how difficult it is to stay with organisations as they find their own way forward. So many organisations will demand that we take the expert role and tell them what to do, provide them with answers that work. There is a great thirst for answers: what is the latest fad, is it 360 degree feedback, outward bound leadership courses, experiential groups, total quality management? It is easy to get caught into that way of thinking: if it is the latest idea it must be good. Organisations, like individuals, have the answers within but never go there – they go for outsiders and outside. Getting organisations to stop and reflect on what is happening to them is amazingly difficult. They don't want to: they want someone to give them the answer, the way forward. That's why they need supervisors who will stay with them as they struggle and work through and come up with their own answers. Certainly, supervisors can make suggestions and recommendations but primarily their job is to facilitate reflection on professional practice and review how values are held and implemented. Bond and Holland (1998) put it well: 'Clinical supervision provides a route to developing and maintaining emotionally healthier individuals in an emotionally healthier culture.' (p.13). Part of that process is to engage in what is called reflectiveness or 'manufactured uncertainty', creating the environment where we make ourselves uncertain as a way of learning. Doing that for our organisations provides a tremendous vehicle for growth and for autonomy.

2. Questioning the myth that the movement is always good

In organisations, there is a strange belief that as long as there is movement there is life. Something happening is better than nothing happening. Noer (1997) has a very graphic image of a modern organisation where clearly movement and action are not harnessed to what is good for the organisation:

> First we decide we are going north and we get on a motorway and drive like hell – at a hundred miles an hour. Then we come to an intersection and we decide to head east and we barrel off in that direction, but that doesn't seem to get us anywhere so we turn around and speed back west, and finally we decide to go back to basics and head south again as fast as we can drive! All the while we are debating who should steer as we watch the petrol gauge moving towards empty. (p.11)

Our task, as supervisors, is to stop the movement in order to review where the organisation is going. Supervision is 'time out' from movement to see what the movement is all about; why have we chosen to go in this direction, is it congruent with our values, is it movement that will help us in the long term? Moore (1992) says that the job of the counsellor is to befriend what the client wants to throw away: 'to look with special attention and openness at what the individual rejects, and then to speak favourably for the rejected element' (p.16). Not bad advice for the supervisor in the organisation. Many organisations want to 'get rid of' without thinking through what they are rejecting or the value to the organisation of what they are throwing out. The whole process of downsizing (or rightsizing as it has been renamed) can result in more harm than good. The research on downsizing and survivor sickness syndrome (what happens to those left behind after downsizing) indicates that more attention should be paid to what is being let go or rejected (Noer 1993; Sahdev and Vinnicombe 1997).

Covey (1989) picks up the movement theme in his writings and produces an image of an organisation as a body moving through the jungle, workers hacking away at the undergrowth, middle managers preparing rotas, making sure their machetes are sharp, workers resting. Where, he asks, are the leaders? Up trees, shouting, 'right direction' or 'we're going the wrong way'. Our job as supervisors is to help get the leaders back up the trees so that the organisation is going, and seen to be going, in the right direction.

The anxiety of organisations forces them to seek guides and guideposts to ease the pain of the journey. Supervision holds anxiety long enough to learn its lessons. An old saying 'an organism in pain keeps moving' is one well known to supervisors. They know when individuals, or organisations stop, the pain comes through. They also know that in the pain is a message, a communication, that, if listened to, gives insight and ways forward. The supervisory task is to help stop the organisation so that it can get in touch with, not just its pain, but its spirit and values. Then we move, with them, to action. It is worth remembering the organisational conundrum concerning the five frogs that sat on a log: four decided to jump into the pond, so how many frogs are now on the log? Five, of course. Why? Because, in organisations, there is no connection between deciding to do something and doing it. As one manager said, 'in our company we don't have human beings, we have human doings'.

As supervisors, we help organisations stop and reflect on what Sell (1999) calls: 'ideas, concepts, opinions, attitudes, moods, thoughts, emotions, human relationships, co-operation, questions of overcoming conflicts, of motivation, loyalties' (p.5). These are not soft skills or soft facts in the working world: 'The most difficult facts in human systems are what simple minds tend to call soft issues.' (Guntern, quoted in Sell 1999, p.5.)

3. Understanding the language of organisations

The words in organisations are important: people can be very frightened if the language we use suggests or hints that they are in need of personal counselling. To talk about mentoring, executive coaching, personal and professional development, organisational efficiency and effectiveness or personal effectiveness is acceptable. It may sound trite but as counsellors and supervisors we know that language carries great weight. The very people who have been shamed and humiliated with language are the ones we are helping heal with new and different words. Preparing for some training with a bank that was making 200 people redundant I mentioned calling the programme 'Giving Bad News'. Personnel were horrified and asked if the title could be changed to 'Notifier Training' and if it could provide them with straightforward 'Steps on how to deal with the separation interview'. The language used is incredible: it is often a way of avoiding the harsh realities behind the words. A recent series of 'Why did the chicken cross the road?' responses on the Internet put this well. The caricature from Anderson Consulting (with apologies) was:

> Deregulation on the chicken's side of the road was threatening its dominant market position. The chicken was faced with significant challenges to create and develop the competencies required for the newly competitive market. Andersen Consulting, in a partnering relationship with the client, helped the chicken by rethinking its physical distribution strategy and implementing processes. Using the Poultry Integration Model (PIM) Andersen consultants helped the chicken use its skills, methodologies, knowledge capital and experiences to align the chicken's people, processes and technology in support of its overall strategy within a Program management framework. Andersen Consulting convened a diverse cross-spectrum of road analysts and best chickens along with Andersen consultants with deep skills in the transportation industry to engage in a two day itinerary of meetings in order to leverage their personal knowledge capital, both tacit and explicit, and to enable them to synergise with each other in order to achieve the implicit goals of delivering and successfully architecting and implementing an enterprise-wide value framework across the continuum of poultry cross-median processes.

Organisations are terrified of giving the wrong message so continually avoid harsh realities by re-naming experiences. Recently, the whole area of downsizing, re-engineering or rightsizing (the more recent term) has been over taken with 'decruiting'. So rather than lay-offs, redundancies, sacking (all terribly negative) we decruit rather than recruit. Reading between the lines of organisational-speak is a skill: *The Guardian* (31 July 1999) had a translation of the real meaning of terms used in the City:

> exceptionally well qualified – has made no major blunders yet
>
> active socially – drinks a lot
>
> family is actively social – partner drinks a lot too
>
> quick thinking – offers plausible excuses
>
> exceptionally good judgement – lucky
>
> has leadership qualities – is tall or has a loud voice
>
> loyal – can't get a job anywhere else
>
> work is first priority – too ugly to get a date.

Language is very important and we can easily use communication as a way of avoiding communication. As supervisors, we understand the importance of words as destructive and as healing, as communication and as avoidance of communication, as facing reality or ignoring it. Can we help organisations find the words that express where they are and where they want to go, to face the realities of what are happening and words that engender hope for the future?

4. Working with the emotional organisation (or the emotions within the organisation)

Within organisations, there is often a great fear of the emotional and of the language of feeling. If there is anything to be learnt from working within organisations it is that they are so frightened of the emotional side that they often collude to believe it does not exist. High level executives are thrown by simple emotions, and that is why they need us as supervisors. There is a tendency to consider everything as rational and if when they get the rational right all else will follow automatically. In training courses, in management, in dealing with people-issues in organisations, the difficulty is to get people thinking emotionally as well as rationally. Many problems within organisations that emerge from areas such as performance management, appraisal, feedback, personal effectiveness, stress management and so on are about working with the emotional side. Supervisors know about emotions and how important they are.

Organisations are wonderful places for privatising emotions. They do it excellently, and individuals join them in doing it. They re-locate feelings and re-name them. Hochschild (1983) coined the phrase 'emotional labour' to show how employees often sell their emotions as well as their 'physical labour' to organisations. Once done, the modern organisation relieves us of the responsibility of having to feel and re-invents our experience for us. It tells us we are responsible for feeling stressed, or depressed, or anxious, or worried or whatever. While laying no claims to supervision expertise, Clint Eastwood discovers this in one of his films and puts it crudely as: 'Don't piss down my back and tell me it's raining'.

It is often the shadow side of the organisation with which we work (Egan 1994). The shadow side of organisations is the arational, the irrational, the emotional and the imaginative. Not necessarily the bad or evil part but the other side: the uncontrolled side. When we ignore it in organisations it always comes back to haunt us: if we stay only with control and reason and sense and sensibility and seriousness and adult, the shadow side has its revenge. People forget who they are: they move into individualism, they become unconnected and work dies and the job becomes more important than life.

It's not that we are unaware of the other side: it's more that we fear it. As Briskin (1998) points out, we must face fears and monsters or they overcome us. When the organisation cannot accept its own shadow-side then it asks people to individualise it and punishes them without looking at the collective shadow and collective responsibility. We build in more repressive policies, bigger prisons. We become obsessed with what we have repressed, as Freud once said, and that obsession emerges in all sorts of ways: physical illnesses, incapacitating stress, deep conflicts in factions in the organisation, unhealthy relationships, individualism, inappropriate sexual contacts. Working with organisations means working with the collective shadow side, not to get rid of it, but to integrate it and use it as a guide (Page 1999). Good supervisors know about integration.

Integrating emotions in organisations inevitably means turning to the subject of men. Most managers are men, most executives are men. Men are not doing well today in the relationship and intimacy journey, what is often referred to as 'the soft skills'. Jourard writes:

> Men are difficult to love. If a man is reluctant to make himself known to another person, even to his spouse because it is not manly to be psychologically naked, then it follows that men will be difficult to love. That is, it will be difficult for a woman or another man to know the immediate present state of the man's self and his needs will thereby go unmet. Some men are so skilled at dissembling, at seeming, that even their wives will not know when they are lonely, bored, anxious, in pain, thwarted, hungering for affection etc. And the man, blocked by pride, dare not disclose his despair or need. The fear of intimacy has held men in terrible isolation and loneliness.

Men are desperately in need of help with relationships. Some statistics seem to indicate the difficulty men have with emotions and emotional life (from *Observer Magazine*, 20 June 1999):

- Men live on average six years less then women.
- Men routinely fail at close relationships (70 per cent of divorces are initiated by women)
- 90 per cent of convicted acts of violence are carried out by men.
- In school, 90 per cent of children with behaviour problems are boys.
- Men make up 95 per cent of inmates in gaols.
- The leading cause of death amongst men between 12 and 60 is self-inflected death. In 1996 in Britain there were 6000 suicides (over 75 per cent by men). There has been a 71 per cent increase in suicide amongst young men in the past 10 years: they are now three times as likely to kill themselves as women are.
- Boys aged 10 to 15 are three times more likely to be involved in violent crime than girls, and 10 times as likely to be involved in drug offences.
- Men are more likely than women to commit drug offences.
- 50 per cent of men between 14 and 25 admit committing an offence.
- 51 per cent of girls attain five or more A–C grade levels at GCSE level compared to 41 per cent of boys.

- Men usually attack certain problems by using only one side of their brain, while women use both sides.
- Four times as many girls call Childline as boys but whey they call, boys tend to report more severe problems.
- Men are three times more likely to be dependent on alcohol than women.
- Six million men drink more than the recommended weekly limit of 21 units compared with one million women who exceed their weekly limit of 14 units.
- In the past five years 21 per cent of men have been working longer hours, compared with 13 per cent of women.

Whether it can be argued that modern society is more 'emotionally disturbed' or not, it does seem that organisations need more help in emotional literacy.

5. Remaining neutral (organisations as collusive places)

Collusion and neutrality are twin themes in organisations. The most difficult of skills for supervisors is remaining neutral when there is pressure to take sides. The result is that many within organisations are either on the side of the individual against the organisation or on the side of the organisation against the individuals. Harvey (1988) has written eloquently on the issue of bystanders and collusion within the organisation pointing out that it is agreement that is often the problem. Organisations need more disagreement and less collusion to agree. He has two very powerful essays in his book called, 'Eichmann in the organization' and 'Organizations as phrog farms'. In the former he takes Eichmann as an example of what is common practice in many organisations – losing our sense of ourselves and colluding with all sorts of inhumane and horrible practices, doing deals that suit no-one in the long run and eventually turning into phrogs (he uses this word instead of 'frogs'), the subject of the second chapter. He warns about it graphically:

> There is a myth amongst phrogs that kissing another phrog turns that phrog into a prince. I think it should be noted that, in general, kissing a phrog only produces skin irritations. For those who decide to kiss anyway, I think that they should realise that in all the fog in the swamp, it is very difficult to determine which way a phrog is facing. (p.41)

The task facing counsellors and supervisors in organisations is to create the kinds of healthy relationships that don't end up as collusive, unhealthily competitive, or dependent so that the good of the organization can come to the top of the agenda. Remaining neutral, not bystanding or colluding, is a supervisor skill well worth cultivating. Petruska Clarkson (1996) has outlined some of the characteristics of bystander behaviour:

- something seems wrong in a situation
- the person is aware of it
- they do not actively take responsibility for their part in maintaining the problem or preventing its resolution ...
- they claim they could not have acted otherwise
- it is based on minimising their capacity for autonomy, intimacy and potency in the world. (p.54)

She has also articulated some of the statements made by bystanders (Clarkson 1996):

it is none of my business

the situation is more complex than it seems

I do not have all the information/am not qualified to deal with this

I don't want to get burned again

I want to remain neutral

I'm only telling the truth as I see it

I'm just following orders

my contribution won't make much difference

they brought it on themselves

I don't want to rock the boat. (pp.56–58)

Supervisors help organisations take responsibility to look at how agreement and disagreement are handled, how conflict resolution and mediation take place and how to build the kinds of relationships that are adult.

6. Focusing on what is good for the organisation

Who really cares for the organisation? Who looks after its needs? The agenda of the organisation, that is, the needs of the organisation, are quite often neglected as the needs of the individuals within the organisation are met. It could well be the job of management to do that, just as it is the job of parents to look after the family. We know that sometimes parents are not able, or choose not, to look after their families: their own needs, their own compulsions, their own unrealistic perceptions sometimes take over and the family suffers. Individual needs may well be met but the organisation, as a whole, suffers.

It is often surprising how many people, especially those in the 'people' or helping side of the company, ally themselves with the individual against the organisation. Instead of using what they are good at with individual work with the organisation, counsellors do the opposite. As they turn from the individual to meet the organisation they change, they become someone else. They become critical, not of their clients, but of their organisation. They forget about empathy, relationship, the agenda of the client, going at the pace of the client, not giving answers that clients can come to themselves, not imposing their own values and:

- they see the faults, the gaps
- they go out to educate
- they fight the organisation
- they keep distance from it
- they don't relate to it
- they don't see the emotional sides of the system.

In other words they work through their agenda, not the agenda of the organisation and as Dorothy Rowe (1990) once remarked, 'the most dangerous people are always those who know what is best for others' (p.17).

As supervisors we try to help individuals do to the organisation what they do to their individual employees. We do not go with the answers, we do not go to educate, or fight, or change, or with our own agenda when we see individual clients. We go to be with, to help them reflect and find their answers and their way through. We go to accept, to understand, to be patient with, to pace, to relate to, to work with, to challenge, to touch the emotions. We follow their agenda, not our own. Why not the same with organisations, allowing their agendas to become foremost?

7. Focusing on the individual within the organisation

First, and it is by no means a novel idea, is that organisations get what they expect. Expect the minimum from employees and don't be surprised when that is what they give. 'Feedforward' is a term being used to indicate how we give feedback in anticipation of behaviour and then those to whom we gave the feedback conveniently live up to expectations. McGregor's (1960) work on Theory X and Theory Y (our understanding of human nature) despite being updated and restated by Pfeffer (1994) is still a long way from being believed. Both Pfeffer's books (*Competitive Advantage Through People*, 1994, and *The Human Equation*, 1998) argue solidly (as did McGregor) that people truly are the best resources and best assets in an organisation. Do organisations really, really believe that? Hardly. But we do as supervisors: our focus is on the person or the person within the organisation. We believe in personhood and if the person is treated right they become what they can become.

Second, employees treat others as they have been treated. There is a cascade effect in how people deal with others and by and large, they do to others what has been done to them. Hampton-Turner (1994) does a masterly job in showing how the principle of caring for employees pays dividends. He concludes:

> It was found in a major study of a US bank that the relationship between the bank's service staff and its customers was repeated in the relationship between supervisors and service staff and was repeated in the relationship between top management and supervisors. It is probable, though the research did not go that far, that the pattern was repeated again between the HQ of the bank and its branches. (p.15)

The bottom line for managers is: employees will treat the customer as you treat employees. This is parallel process – how well we know, as supervisors, how what happens in one system ends up in another; how what supervisors do to supervisees is often, in turn, done to clients and vice versa.

Third, we can no longer view the performance of employees as an isolated event that occurs because of their own internal abilities; it is connected to organisational culture, to motivation, to relationships at work and home. Much employee behaviour is a response to the situation in which employees find themselves; it is not bad-mindedness, poor attitudes, or the need for training. Organisations rarely think of human behaviour as connected to the organisation. 'Perhaps he or she is acting that way because of the way you are treating them' is a big statement for an organisation to hear. They still think in terms of, 'take them out, sort them out and sent them back repaired'.

Applying supervision to organisations

The European Association for Supervision has widened the concept of supervision from simply clinical work and comments that:

> In this way supervision is making an important contribution to the development of quality in organisations and their services through: individual supervision, group supervision, team supervision, coaching. Supervision is contributing essentially to learning organisations and will lead into processes of team development and organisational development. (ANSE, undated).

While there are a number of ways in which supervisors can be involved in supervision/consultation within organisations, four of these are:

1. Individual supervision of people who work within organisations: work with managers, with directors, with HR and personnel. Desperate for

supervision: the principles of how to work as a supervisor in this context have been outlined elsewhere (Carroll 1999).

2. Supervising teams and groups within organisations (see Lammers 1999 and Proctor 2000, in press, for ideas in this area).
3. Supervising executive teams.
4. Supervising organisations themselves (Noer 1993).

Space does not permit looking in more detail at these four areas of supervision within organisations. However, there is a set of skills brought by supervisors to these areas within organisational settings:

- process skills: reflection in depth, going beneath the surface and helping organisations get in touch with their own processes
- healthy relationships: facilitating and modelling helpful and adult relationships within the organisation
- connections skills: helping organisations make connections within the organisation and outside it
- emotions: how to deal with the emotional side of the organisation
- pain: staying with, listening to and learning from the pain-communication at the various levels of the organisation
- agenda focus: how to work with the agenda of the organisation (Carroll 1998)
- facilitating change: supervising the organisation as it learns how to prepare for, introduce and sustain effective change.

My argument in this chapter is that supervisors are one of the few groups of professionals who have these sets of skills so desperately needed by organisations.

Conclusion

Changing our mindsets to work, as supervisors, within organisations involves a movement between two mentalities:

- from individual thinking to organisational thinking
- from individual assessment to assessment in a context
- from interpersonal relationships to systems relations
- from uni-role involvement to multi-role involvement
- from personal accountability to organisational accountability
- from non-evaluation to evaluation
- from single intervention to organisational intervention
- from personal change to organisational change.

Organisations are amazing places to work: they are full of idealism and despair, they desperately seek change and they hate change, they create health and support amazing regression, they ask for feedback and kill when they are told what they do not want to hear, they are filled with great co-operation and incredible collusion. They are never dull. And they need supervision – badly.

References

Association for National Organisations for Supervision in Europe (ANSE) (undated) *Supervision in Europe.* Berne: ANSE Publication.

Berridge, J., Cooper, C. L. and Highley-Marchington, C. (1997) *Employee Assistance Programmes and Workplace Counselling.* Chichester: Wiley.

Bond, M. and Holland, S. (1998) *Skills of Clinical Supervision for Nurses.* Buckingham: Open University Press.

Briskin, A. (1998) *The Stirring of Soul in the Workplace.* San Francisco, CA: Berrett-Koehler.

Carroll, M. (1998) 'The agenda of the organisation.' *Occupational Medicine 46,* 6, 411–412.

Carroll, M. (1999) 'Supervision in workplace counselling.' In M. Carroll and E. Holloway (eds) *Counselling Supervision in Context.* London: Sage.

Clarkson, P. (1996) *The Bystander.* London: Whurr Publications.

Covey, S. (1989) *The Seven Habits of Highly Effective People.* London: Simon and Schuster.

Egan, G. (1994) *Working the Shadow-Side: A Guide to Positive Behind-the-Scenes Management.* San Francisco, CA.: Jossey-Bass.

Hampton-Turner, C. (1994) *Corporate Culture.* London: Piatkus.

Harvey, J. (1988) *The Abilene Paradox and other Meditations on Management.* San Francisco, CA: Jossey-Bass.

Hochschild, A.R. (1983) *The Managed Heart: Commercialisation of Human Feeling.* Berkeley, CA: University of California Press.

Lammers, W. (1999) 'Training in group and team supervision.' In E. Holloway and M. Carroll (eds) *Training Counselling Supervisors: Strategies, Methods and Techniques.* London: Sage.

McGregor, D. (1960) *The Human Side of Enterprise.* New York, NY: Mc Graw-Hill.

Moore, T. (1992) *Care of the Soul.* London: Piatkus.

Noer, D. (1997) *Breaking Free: A Prescription for Personal and Organizational Change.* San Francisco, CA: Jossey-Bass.

Noer, D. (1993) *Healing the Wounds: Overcoming the Trauma of Layoffs and Revitalising Downsized Organizations.* San Francisco, CA: Jossey-Bass.

Page, S. (1999) *The Shadow and the Counsellor.* London: Routledge.

Pfeffer, J. (1994) *Competitive Advantage through People.* Boston, MA: Harvard University Press.

Pfeffer, J. (1998) *The Human Equation.* Boston, MA: Harvard University Press.

Pilgrim, D. (1997) *Psychotherapy and Society.* London: Sage.

Proctor, B. (2000) *Group Supervision.* London: Sage.

Rowe, D. (1990) 'Foreword.' In J. Masson *Against Therapy.* London: Fontana.

Sahdev, K. and Vinnicombe, S. (1997) *Downsizing and Survivor Syndrome: A Study of HR's Perception of Survivors' Responses.* Bedford: Cranfield School of Management.

Sell, M. (1999) 'The supervisor – a professional identity.' *ID: EAS,* July, 3–7.

Chapter 5

Integrative Supervision

Art and Science

Julie Hewson

Introduction

This chapter has been a challenge for me, not least in endeavouring to put into a succinct way something that as a storyteller rather than a writer I could do better in dialogue. I have noticed that the language, sentence structure and phraseology is markedly different when I write from the scientific as opposed to the artistic side of the subject. In *being* it, I believe I integrate the two easily and seamlessly; in writing I still think I have some way to go to achieve that integration in the written word. So, as you read this chapter, bear with me in my attempts to find the language of both, and know that if we were together in a room, the dance between the two arenas in dialogue could be a delight.

Supervision is an art and a science, a relationship and a knowledge base, an encouraging and supportive process as well as a monitoring one. The art of supervision is the ability to create a safe space, a relationship where the re-creation of natural curiosity and observation can be validated and enhanced. Supervision is the development of trust and respect, and the willingness to meet in an encounter of mutuality and mentorship. It requires sensitivity to the potential emergence of shame, needing an eye and an expertise not only to the subject matter but also in how to enhance the learning environment. The artistry of supervision has at it service at least five potential relationships:

- the working alliance
- the I–Thou relationship
- the transference – countertransference relationship (with the client)
- the developmentally needed reparative relationship (in supervision this is likely to be educative)
- the transpersonal relationship (Clarkson 1995).

The artistry in supervision is the combination of managing an educative and assessing/monitoring role with therapeutic skill. This, inevitably, revolves around managing the supervisory relationship. Described as 'a working alliance between a supervisor and a counsellor' (Inskipp and Proctor 1993), the supervisory relationship may, at first sight, resemble the therapeutic alliance. It certainly is at its best a relationship that includes many of the core conditions and therapeutic elements belonging to counselling and psychotherapy but its focus and outcome is entirely different. To manage such a subtle relationship is an art. When this balancing act fails, students have reported feeling shamed and their boundaries violated (Hewson 2000; Sweeney 1997).

While endeavouring to empower supervisees in their development, supervision is an asymmetrical or unequal relationship. Holloway (1998) has reviewed the concept of power in supervision, describing it as involving two dimensions: 'power over' and 'power with'. In the 'power over' role supervisors have to evaluate supervisees, be 'gatekeepers of the profession' and be accountable to clients, training courses and the public in general. In 'power with' supervisors are required to empower supervisees to take on the mantle of skills and knowledge needed for their roles as counsellors and be responsible for themselves. Putting together the two areas of engagement and power she outlines a matrix depicted in Figure 5.1.

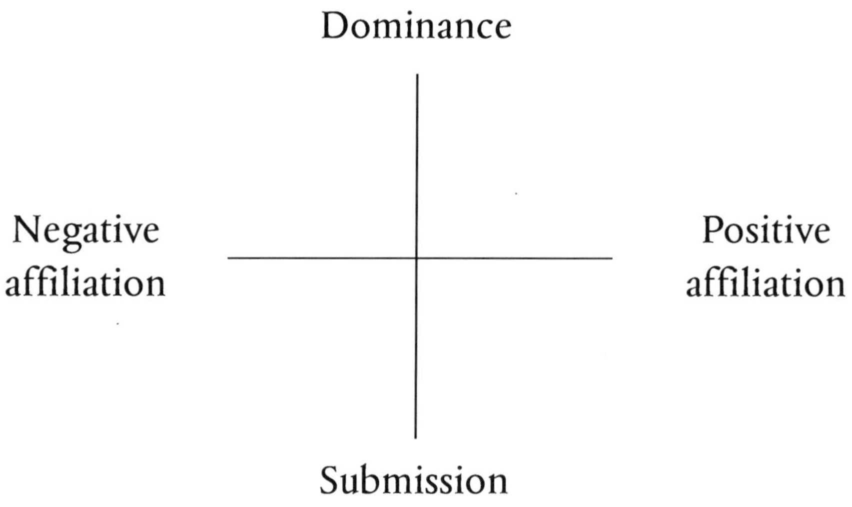

Figure 5:1: Engagement and power in supervision (Holloway 1998). Reprinted with the kind permission of Elizabeth Holloway.

In her research she asked supervisees, at different stages of training development, about their experience of supervision. Not surprisingly, the issue of power emerged frequently in quotations such as 'The supervisor has more authority'. Ways in which the supervisory relationship could be made more mutual were:

- contracting for honest, positive and critically constructive feedback for and from both supervisor and supervisee and
- providing a clear description of evaluation criteria and procedures.

Figure 5.2 demonstrates the range of factors and the significance of the collaborative relationship.

Holloway (1998) has also highlighted factors that militate against the inequalities of power in supervision. These included situations where a supervisee

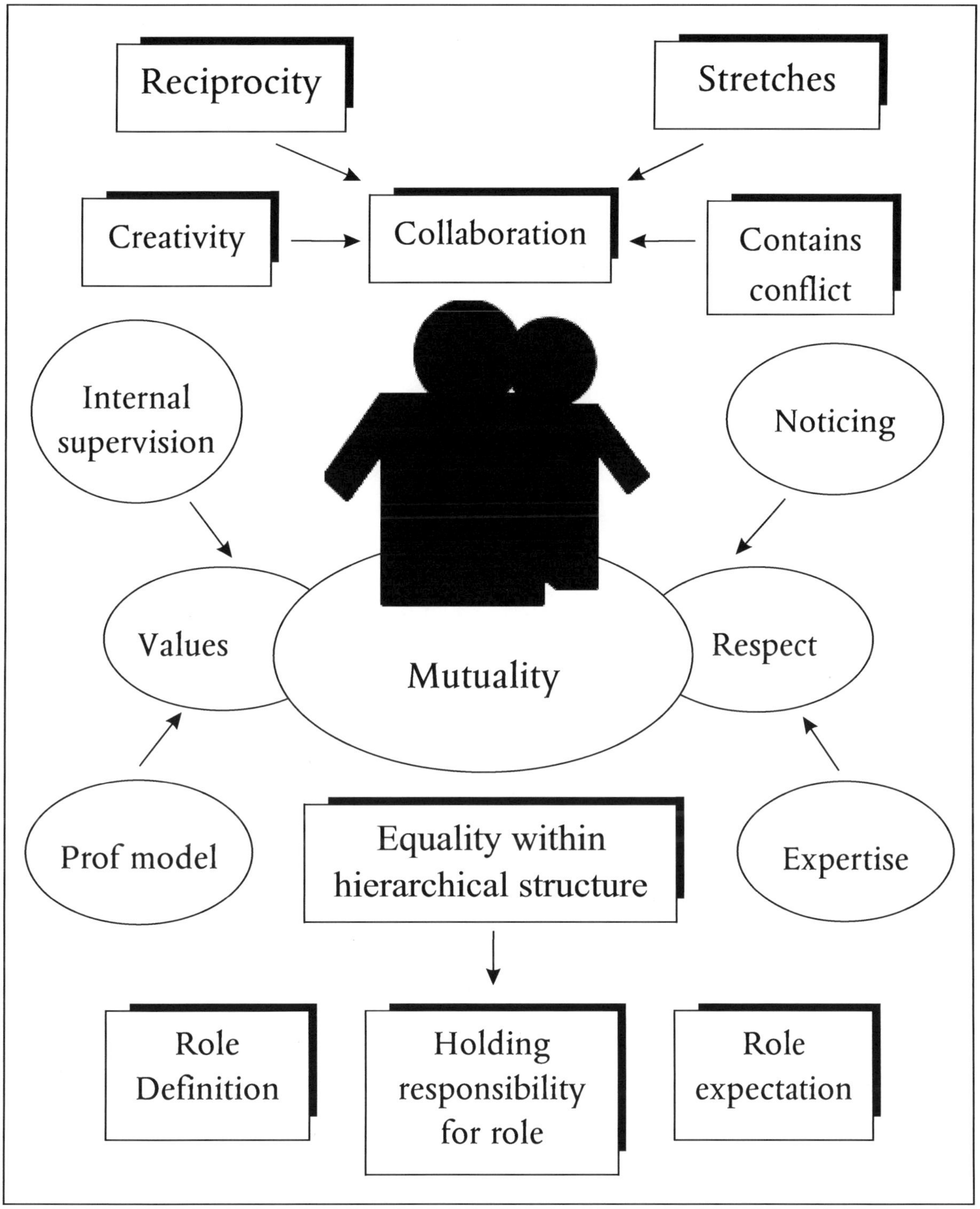

Figure 5.2: Through the eyes of the supervisee (Holloway 1998). Reprinted with the kind permission of Elizabeth Holloway.

is able to change supervisor, where the supervisee is paying for supervision and is therefore the customer, and supervisory arrangements where roles and criteria are clarified at the outset.

Factors that precipitated problems in supervisory relationships especially around issues of power included:

- hierarchical structures within organisations where the supervisee feels they have no choice of supervisor and
- where a supervisor has multiple roles in relation to the supervisee.

This latter example has been addressed by social services in Devon in the last five years, where line-management and case supervision are now conducted by different people.

Another factor that brings together the strands of the supervisory relationship, power differentials and the art and science of managing tasks, functions and relationships is the developmental stage of supervisees. Since supervision is an interpersonal container for a range of professional tasks including pedagogy, analysis, consultation, personal growth and awareness, and the development of skills, it is clear that supervisees move through stages of development in respect of these areas. Hence, the needs of novice supervisees will be different from the needs of supervisees at intermediate and advanced levels. Novices often start questions with 'Tell me about ...', an indicator that they are looking for answers and a recognition of themselves in the counselling process (Holloway 1998). They also report needing their past professional skills acknowledged and efforts of good work recognised. The supervisee needs, at this stage, to be seen for who they are without being blemished or judged. When the supervisory relationship failed during this period of development, it was judged to have failed in terms of a lack of mutuality leading to dismay and withdrawal.

Intermediate and advanced supervisees, on the other hand, seem more concerned with whether the supervisor's expertise warranted respect. Several reported watching the supervisor as a professional counsellor and assessing whether they were a good role model.

Thus it is clear that there is a developmental progression in the development of professionals which is reflected in the supervisory process as well as in its tasks and functions (Carroll 1996; Holloway 1995; Stoltenberg and Delworth 1987). A key issue here is that of dealing with the polarities of 'cosiness and stretching' within the provision of 'a nest of mutual respect' (Holloway 1998). If there is not enough stretching the supervisee can feel professionally deadened. 'It was becoming too cosy' was one reported phrase. Thus, there is a sense of reciprocal responsibility in the supervisory relationship.

The science of supervision

The science of supervision begins with classification, naming, grouping and discovering the linear logical deductive processes within the supervisory process, a sort of what has led to what. This is a procedure of looking for evidence to support an intuitive hunch. It requires the supervisor and supervisee to link the phenomenological experiences of working with patients and clients with observable patterns, clusters of traits, predictable outcomes and assessment of probabilities.

There are three models that show different aspects of science of supervision (Carroll 1996; Holloway 1995; Irving 1996). The first two have both researched their frameworks academically and yet both present supervision as a form of artistry. Irving has approached it from a scientific position of assessing competencies and finding ways to measure them.

Holloway (1995) takes us through the supervision functions of:

- monitoring and evaluating
- advising and instructing
- modelling
- consulting
- supporting and sharing as a way of addressing the supervisory tasks which are the development and honing of:
- counselling/psychotherapeutic skills
- case conceptualisation
- professional roles
- emotional awareness
- self-evaluation.

All of these involve the clarification of both the role and contract with the supervisor, the awareness of the developmental stage of the supervisee and the agreed range of responsibility of the supervisor.

Carroll (1996) sets out seven generic tasks of supervision, which were discovered through his research of supervisors and supervisees. These are:

- to consult
- to monitor administrative aspects
- to set up a learning relationship
- to teach
- to evaluate
- to monitor professional ethical issues

- to counsel.

The classifications above have given form to what might have been previously seen as a rather ill-defined development out of mastery in a particular field. What both these writers show is that the tasks and functions require other skills and knowledge beyond the original training.

Each of these roles are compatible with a transactional analytic way of working in that the place of teaching and coaching and the sharing of paradigms is part of the therapeutic process, engaging the client to become the other therapist in the room. This involves being able to stand back and comment on patterns and outcomes, as well as make sense of the reasons behind these. In addition to these overall tasks, Irving (1995) has formulated a set of competencies that transactional analysts can employ to assess the tasks and functions of supervision. As these are too lengthy to include here, a few examples of these competencies will give a flavour. The ones here are some expected of therapists and monitored by supervisors:

> 'The therapist knows and monitors own internal world and response during psychotherapy and prevents own difficulties from interfering with understanding of the client.'
>
> 'The therapist differentiates own feelings from clients' feelings as evidenced by crossed transactions.'
>
> 'The therapist can identify when the client has developed their own inner resources to complete the therapy.'
>
> 'Therapists makes clear the nature and extent of confidentiality as circumscribed by law, individual and/or agency culture and stance and therapeutic context.'

The art and the science of supervision

One model that addresses the connections between the art and science of supervision is the seven-level model of Clarkson and Lapworth (1992). This model takes seven universes of discourse, each of which has a subtle emphasis on the art, the science or the combination of the two in the particular field to which it is applied.

1. The first is the level of sensation. In supervision it is of the essence to pay attention to physical manifestations, both in the presentation of the client and within the felt experience of the supervisee and the supervisor's countertransference response. Part of the supervisor's role is to ensure that there is a balance of attention in this domain and that basic medical information is noted, including medication, family history of illnesses and any recurring 'accidents'. An exercise to access this

universe is to ascertain where on a physiological level the client impacts on the supervisee. Having located the place speak from it, for example, I am Amanda's throat and I am aware of feeling choked whenever my client speaks of her childhood even though she reports the events without emotion.

2. The second is the level of awareness and emotion, the realm of intuition. This universe is where hunches are born, a knowing sometimes without knowing why. This can include emotions and feelings in response to the client. In Hawkins' and Shohet's (1989) model of the six-eyed supervisor this is the one where the focus is on the relationship between client and practitioner. This is often where an intuitive feeling is acted out in the relationship. An exercise to access this level can be to ask the supervisee to choose an animal that might represent the client and speak as that animal. This was found to be very effective by a Czech supervisee who was having difficulties in her multi-disciplinary team following a change in organisational structure. The supervisee was a highly educated and cerebral person and found that choosing and as it were becoming each of the animals in her team gave her a new insight into the internal and external processes of each and her unconscious understanding of them. The supervisee actually moved and imitated the way such a creature might sound if it had speech.

3. The third level is the nominative. This leads us into the arena of naming and labelling, classifying and differentiating. A psychodynamic supervisor or counsellor might place far more emphasis on unconscious motivation than would an existentialist or a cognitive-behaviourist, and frame it in different language. The importance of language and labels is that they provide a vehicle for differentiation of generalisation. Part of the supervisor's role is to enable supervisees to diagnose effectively for the purposes of risk assessment, to name in language what is happening. This may well involve them in studying the psychiatric diagnostic nomenclature of DSMIVR and ICD10 or the use of other methods of assessment. An exercise at this level would be to describe a client in more than one modality or approach, for example from a psychodynamic perspective, a Kelly's construct perspective, a Gestalt and transactional analytic perspective.

4. The fourth level is normative. This realm encompasses ethics, values, professional practice, cultural differences, religion. These may pertain to the client's culture and value system. Issues of race, gender, ethnicity, sexual orientation and religion lie here. This is also true of the

supervisor and the organisational setting in which the work is carried out. Different organisations are based on very different value systems and quite often people assume they are compatible with their own. This is not always the case. This realm begs a range of questions not least relating to the ethics of psychotherapy and counselling as a profession at all. It could be very good practice on a regular basis to question, why am I doing this work at all? What are my values? Do they need reviewing? This is a way of assessing change within practitioners and matching them to changes within the organisations, such as the NHS, the teaching profession as well as psychotherapy and counselling, as well as monitoring for burnout. Many supervisees are commenting on high levels of professional stress because the job they came into the profession to do is no longer there. Take the example of creative teachers being stifled by the national curriculum, and GPs swamped by the enormous numbers of forms that they now have to fill in.

5. The fifth level is that of the rational. So much psychotherapy is based on a quest for meaning that the methodology of how to effect change is sometimes missing. Strategies from cognitive behavioural, cognitive analytic and rational emotive therapies, Kelly's construct theory and transactional analysis all have their contribution to make here. An exercise that would demonstrate this is the three-chair decontamination exercise between three ego-states from transactional analysis. Such a method could be used for the supervisee as well as the client to separate out what feeling thoughts and behaviours are current, archaic or borrowed. There are many strategies and techniques within cognitive analytic therapy, CBT, RET and Kelly's construct theory.

6. The sixth level is that of meaning, of hypothesis, of storyline. This is the level where theories are developed based on data collected at the other levels. There are developmental models, drive models, relational models, models based on the interface between the intrapsychic and the interpersonal, models based on social psychology, on existential human dilemmas and theories based on the personal and collective unconscious. The plurality of models sometimes poses questions on the match of supervisor to supervisee at different stages in the supervisee's development. There are also questions to be raised relating to making the client fit the model rather than the model being in the service of the client. The very nature of some theoretical constructs can pathologise where no pathology exists. This level also encompasses the level of metaphor, as meaning can be derived in this way and does give the supervisor the opportunity to literally employ art in the supervisory

process, through drawing, analogy, poetry, puppetry and even the use of sand tray work. All this depends on a number of factors, not least the level of knowledge and training of the supervisor and the clear demarcation of the boundary between supervision and personal therapy. My research suggests that the violation of this boundary is one of the key areas of distress for supervisees.

7. The seventh level is that of the transpersonal where mysticism and spirituality, universality and compassion are most fully expressed. As a supervisor it is important to be alert to the openness of the supervisee to such expressions of the psyche. Some clients come soul-sick rather than heart-sick. To be aware of the significance of this sphere in our lives, which for many is all-encompassing and for others seems absent, is of critical importance. There are those clients and supervisees who are at an existential or spiritual crossroads, who need the sanctuary of a place and a relationship to find their way again. To miss the significance of this is to be in danger of pathologising the client, reducing all symptoms to early developmental issues or irrational self statements. The art of supervision requires us to refresh our own souls or spirit, whatever we wish to call this part of ourselves, in music, art, laughter, nature, meditation and joy. As supervisors this helps us refresh our vision, our hearing, our wonder and awe at the miraculous qualities our patients, clients and supervisees present. There is, for me, a never-ending amazement at the dignity and resourcefulness of many who are under terrible adversity as well as the misery and degradation that we as humans perpetrate and suffer.

Conclusion

Ken Wilbur (1998) distinguishes between differentiated and undifferentiated approaches to our relationship with the world. Differentiated relates to modernism, science, a tendency towards reductionism, a sense of modern alienation. Undifferentiated approaches were alive in pre-modern cultures, where there was no separation between art, morals and science. This had its own difficulties, for example, Galileo being charged with heresy for his scientific beliefs; and there was a place for the souls and spirit and a sense of the great chain of being. The areas of focus in human discovery have been of matter, life, mind, soul and spirit, and Wilbur equates each of these areas with the realm of study of physics, biology, psychology, theology and mysticism respectively. In supervision we are faced with the challenge of how to integrate these two strands, these two traditions. Do we go for epistemological pluralism and see the world with the 'eye of the flesh' (science) 'the eye of the mind' (logic) and/or the 'eye of contemplation' (gnosis). Plotinus (in Wilbur 1998, p.18) saw that there were many levels of abstraction: matter, life, sensation, perception, impulse, images, concepts, logical faculty, creative reason and world soul; in addition, the intuitive NOUS and the one absolute Godhead. Wilbur (1998) mourns the loss in modern times of the eye of the contemplative and the eye of the spirit.

In our world we have all these strands and more, and our work as individuals is to weave them into a carpet of our own making, with the colours we were given or have found. Supervision is a role and a professional oasis where some of these can be addressed in relation to helping each other find a path with a heart and to revert to the previous analogy, unravel the tangles from attempts at rugs and tapestries in the past.

Supervision is a complex, technical, sensitive and fairly new area of facilitating professional competence. It has more in common with education than counselling, but still employs many of the skills and techniques from psychotherapy and counselling, such as the ability to build a safe relationship, to use clear listening skills, to support and confront, and manage both support and challenge. It therefore has to be more than a series of models and methods and more than a holding supportive relationship in which to learn. It is the combination of strategic thinking and a sensitive enabling/mentoring relationship that will make the balance of art and science, one that will be in the service of supervisees and clients. The very nature of the change of language throughout this chapter shows the balancing act and dance that can go on between the different realms.

Science requires a sound theoretical framework or frameworks against which to test observations. Artistry, on the other hand, is the balance of sensitivity and awareness to adult learners working with vulnerable people in a way that often leaves them open to unexpectedly high levels of emotional impact. This requires more than skill, it goes beyond that which can be taught, it is the integration of personal qualities and knowledge: at its best it is the combination of wisdom and understanding.

References

Carroll, M. (1996) *Counselling Supervision: Theory, Skills and Practice.* London: Cassell.

Clarkson, P. (1995) *The Therapeutic Relationship.* London: Whurr.

Clarkson, P. and Lapworth, P. (1992) 'Systemic integrative psychotherapy.' In W. Dryden (ed) (1996) *Integrative and Eclectic Psychotherapy: A Handbook.* Buckinghamshire: Open University Press.

Hawkins, P. and Shohet, R. (1989) *Supervision in the Helping Professions.* Milton Keynes: Open University Press.

Hewson J. (2000) Research dissertation in progress. Exeter University.

Holloway, E. (1995) *Clinical Supervision: A Systems Approach.* London: Sage.

Holloway, E. (1998) *Power in the Supervisory Relationship.* Keynote address, British Association of Supervision Practice and Research conference, London, England.

Inskipp, F. and Proctor, B. (1993) *The Art, Craft and Tasks of Counselling Supervision: Part 1: Making the Most of Supervision.* Twickenham: Cascade.

Irving, N. (1995) *Core Competence for Transactional Analysis.* Psychotherapy discussion document.

Stoltenberg, C. D. and Delworth, U. (1987) *Supervising Counselors and Therapists.* San Francisco, CA: Jossey-Bass.

Sweeney, G. (1997) *An Examination of the Processes Underlying Supervision in Occupational Therapy.* Exeter University. With permission.

Wilbur, K. (1998) *The Marriage of Sense and Soul: Integrating Science and Religion.* New York: Random House.

Chapter 6

The Spirituality of Supervision

Michael Carroll

Introduction

Spirituality is becoming a topical subject. Recently it has been connected to the workplace (Thorne 1998), to secular professions (Thorne 1997) and to psychotherapy (West 2000). This chapter will attempt the same connecting process, only the focus and relationship here will be between supervision and spirituality.

Spirituality, like supervision, begins with questions and the quest for truth inevitably leads to questions. Since spirituality and supervision are both concerned with aspects of human behaviour then the first questions concern themselves with destructive human behaviour. Why did groups of people travel to France to support a football team during the World Cup and then systematically tear the place apart and beat up rival fans? Why did a group of white men attack a young black man in East London a few years ago and kill him because he was black? Why do we have yearly carnivals at hot spots in Northern Ireland where confrontation between two branches of the same Christian religion (dictates of which religion are about neighbourliness, love and forgiveness) spar up and often kill one another? What is happening that so many people turn to crime, that our prisons are overflowing, that many streets are unsafe to walk and that all sorts of crimes are perpetrated against women? American citizens, when asked, 'Do you think life will be better for your children that it was for you?' have always answered 'yes'. Until 1988: for the first time a majority said 'no' (Keen 1994). Why do people, myself included, say that they are glad they do not have to start living their lives again and sense that the pressures faced by young people today far exceed what we had to face growing up in the 1960s and 1970s. Why this mistrust of the future?

The answers to the questions above about destructive human behaviour are very complex. It's too easy to say some people are bad, or mad, or deprived, or aggressive or born that way, or emotionally illiterate or whatever. However, might it be possible that all of the people involved in the situations mentioned above (and the examples above could be multiplied and adapted when other countries and societies are reviewed) are *not* in personal supervision. Some of them might be being supervised but not in a chosen, one-to-one or small group supervision where they reflect on life, how they live, what their values are, how they can grow and develop and what is healthy and unhealthy human behaviour. Is it possible that if they were in supervision they might not be involved in these kinds of destructive behaviour? Of course, there are people in clinical supervision who have abused their clients – clearly, being in supervision is no guarantee that a person cannot be destructive in respect of others. But leaving aside the simple fact of being present in supervision, is it possible that adopting a supervisory attitude, viewing supervision as a reflective process that allows participants to think deeply and vulnerably about life and values, work and career, relationships and connections, might make an immense difference in how participants live? There is no scientific evidence that connects the ability and opportunity to reflect on life and the resultant living of a more peaceful, less violent existence. And yet if Socrates could remark wisely that 'the unexamined life is not worth living' there would seem to be some grounds for believing that the more we think about life, work, relationships, leisure and fun, the more chances there are that we will find ourselves in healthier relationships with ourselves, others and our world.

A distinction can be drawn between 'functional supervision', that is, supervision as a technology and a 'philosophy of supervision', that is, supervision as a way of being in much the same way as Rogers talked about counselling as a way of being (Rogers 1980). In its 'functional' mode supervision is something done, applied techniques, strategies and methods used for some purpose. A 'philosophy of supervision' focuses on the 'being of people' and the meaning supervision has for us is almost before anything is done. I remember meeting a carpenter who talked about his profession as a part of himself – it was him, not just a job he did. He saw shapes in wood that only he could see, he visualised the final product before he even took out a chisel. He befriended everything: tools, wood, concepts, ideas, drawings. In many ways that is the ideal for all professions and all jobs: when human beings work they use themselves as the main focus of their work, they infuse themselves into it, they become it; it is them at work, not just work done by them. Their work changes from being a job, or indeed even a career, to becoming an extension of themselves, of who they are. When that does not happen then the spiritual dimension of their work is missing. Because spirituality is about what is being done all the time, not the stuff being done when work is over. It is one of those 'all or nothing' situations: spirituality is in everything or it is in nothing: it's a way of looking at, being with, and connecting to, even imposing on. The spirituality of supervision is the same: it's what people are and how they view life and how they live – that is, supervision as a way of life, supervision as a value system that drives as much personally as it does professionally. Or else it is something that may or may not be connected to who we are, functional supervision.

There is 'religious supervision' and 'spiritual supervision'. There is a distinction between the two as there is between religion and spirituality. In using the term 'spirituality' there is no necessary connection to organised religion, or God, or particular denominational structures. Spirituality may be connected to these but not necessarily so. Many would hold that contemporary religions have lost spirituality rather than represent or mediate it. However, there is little chance of spirituality itself getting lost. Sam Keen (1994) writes:

> Spirituality is in. Millions who have become disillusioned with a secular view of life and are unmoved by established religion in any of its institutional forms are setting out on a quest for something – some missing value, some absent purpose, some new meaning, some presence of the sacred. (p.xix)

Perhaps the 'supervisory life' might be one way of being in touch with what is real, beyond us and still within us, which brings out the best in us.

What happens then, in supervision, is that we learn to live inside-out rather than outside-in (a term coined by Covey 1989). The 'outside-in supervisor', or counsellor or policeman/woman is an expert, a technician who is doing something to someone else. Their task and their work are not necessarily connected to them as a person. The inside-out professional is someone whose job comes from inside. The inside-out supervisor knows that the beginning is always with self, not the other, that no matter how knowledgeable, skilled or competent you are, if you're 'not OK' inside then you won't 'be OK' outside. Covey, in his best selling book, *The Seven Habits of Highly Effective People* (1989), talks to managers about this:

> If I try to use human influence strategies and tactics of how to get other people to do what I want, to work better, to be more motivated, to like me and each other – while my character is fundamentally flawed, marked by duplicity and insincerity – then, in the long run, I cannot be successful. My duplicity will breed distrust and everything I do – even using so called good human relations techniques – will be perceived as manipulative. It simply makes no difference how good the rhetoric or even how good the intentions are: there is little or no trust, there is no foundation for permanent success. (p.21)

That is quite a statement from a management consultant talking about other managers. Where is there talk like that in the city, in the banks, in industry, in business schools, on MBA courses? Where managers gather, is there talk of spirituality, the interior life and getting it right inside yourself before trying to lead or manage others? Emerson's quotation in Covey's book captures the essence of this: 'What you *are* shouts so loudly in my ears that I cannot hear what you say' (p.22). Covey's insight is that the message is not distinct from me: 'You *are* the message' or '*You* are the message'. We are supervision-in-action (supervisors-in-action) rather than functional supervisors. The best principle of education is that individuals learn from what they see rather than from what they hear. We do more readily what is modelled for us rather than what others tell us to do.

Inside-out supervision is about supervision as a way of life. Supervisors live the supervisory life, they don't just do something to others. The values of supervision are the values of life, the position and stance taken, the belief system underlying behaviour. Supervisors supervise themselves first of all before being supervisors to and of others. Living the supervisory life precedes being a supervisor to others in much the same way as spiritual directors have lived and been involved in what they are helping others find and discover for themselves.

In the light of this there are six propositions on the spirituality of the supervisory life to consider:

1. becoming reflective
2. learning, and learning how to learn
3. becoming process oriented
4. establishing healthy relationships
5. learning connectness
6. becoming an interior person.

1. Becoming reflective

Is there a direct proportion and relationship between reflecting on life and perpetrating violence? If life and living are pondered on, thought about, contemplated more, would that increase the chances of being more in harmony with people and reduce chances of hurting or destroying others? Reflecting on life pushes people inwards to know their questions and answers and values and queries and the connections between all these. Reflection can, of course, take place alone, or with others, in groups, in crowds. But reflection is a stance, a position vis-à-vis the world. What does it mean?

Without reflection and contemplation the external becomes what is important. Martin Luther is said to have written, summarily, that a person without spirituality becomes his or her own exterior. Reflection and 'thinking about' creates an opening in the surface world of things, to use O'Donohue's phrase (1997). That is why reflection is so important to life. Not a reflection that is driven by the need to have answers but a reflection that sets out to learn the questions, understanding that there are not always answers and rarely set answers. Not to reflect on life is to live by scripts written by other people, being predetermined. It is to live a co-dependent life, depending on others for answers to questions I don't even ask, and these are not my questions anyway. As the old joke says, 'You know you are co-dependent when you're dying and someone else's life passes in front of your eyes'. The spiritual journey begins when we turn away from our standard answers and turn towards fresh questions. The religious quest is the opposite of the spiritual quest. Keen (1994) captures it well in the distinctions he makes between religion and spirituality:

> One is about answers, the other about questions.
>
> One is well mapped, the other is uncharted.
>
> One is about obedience, the other is about openness, waiting and trust.
>
> One is about repetition, the other is about inventing, creating.
>
> One is about sacred places and objects, the other is about sacred people.
>
> One is about ascending, the other about descending.
>
> One is based on other worlds, the other finds the sacred in life and work.
>
> One is institutional and corporate, the other is individual and communal.
>
> One is about rising above it all, the other is about being immersed in it.

In the light of this distinction supervision can be either religious or spiritual. Supervision based on the religious mode has all the answers, is well mapped, has calls for obedience, and is about sacred ways. Supervision that is spiritual is the opposite: it goes to search, to be with, to think through, to find pathways that last for a while and then these are pathways no more.

The same distinction between religion and spirituality can be applied to organisations, institutions and companies today. They desperately want religion, not spirituality. No one has time to stop and think, there is no right or wrong, there is only what works, now. There is no long-term reflection or planning, only the latest fad that promises the quick fix, the solution. Organisations are desperate for saviours and indeed there are enough saviours around if the price is right; we call them consultants.

Organisations watch their competitors to show them the agenda: they lose their souls and therefore find it hard to become spiritual places; which is not surprising since no one loves them anyway and they remain outside-in organisations rather than inside-out organisations.

Neufeldt (1999) has written very well about reflectivity as the kernel of supervision. She calls it 'focused contemplation' where supervisees think deeply about what has happened so as to discover new learning. She outlines three steps in reflection:

- locus of attention: attend to actions, emotions, thoughts, interactions, processes, organisations
- stance or position: examine in some depth

  critical inquiry

  openness to what is there

  vulnerability
- the use of theory and experience. (pp.94–5)

Supervision of client work uses this kind of reflectivity well. There is no reason why reflectivity cannot be an agenda for a way of life, applying the process above to life and living, to relationships, to work, to leisure, to who we are and what we want to be. Reflectiveness is about changing paradigms as was outlined in the film *Dead Poet's Society* in which Robin Williams gives his pupils a symbol for seeing differently: he asks them to stand up on their desks to get a new view of old things. We see differently when we allow new awarenesses to hit us, to pierce the armour. Was Pascal overstating it when he said that all of humanity's problems stem from man's inability to sit quietly in a room alone? Not to reflect is not to change.

2. Learning, and learning how to learn

The spirituality of supervision is about ongoing learning, learning as a way of life and learning how to learn. Paradigms change all the time and what is most important is often forgotten. We learn and unlearn and relearn and learn again (Carroll 2000) and eventually learn that we know nothing really. As the poet T.S. Eliot once said, we truly come back to the beginning and recognise it for the first time or in the philosopher Kierkegaard's words, 'You live life forward, you understand it backwards'. Knowledge can be accumulated without becoming wise, age is no guarantee against stupidity and being powerful does not necessarily equate with knowing. Learning at the heart of life is a difficult philosophy – it entails being alert for surprises, willing to change, open. So much is missed because the opportunity of being surprised is gone. There is no wonder, amazement, curiosity and uncertainty. The Edinburgh Institute of Contemporary Art had a notice at its entrance, which read:

> As you come into this centre please bring your gallery bag with you: In your gallery bag you will find:
>
> a new pair of eyes: a mind's eye because real eyes are not enough
>
> a new brain
>
> a special camera

lots of questions

a pair of lips (preferably smiling)

a tape measure.

A learning lifestyle is what spirituality is about. Religion is for those who need to know, who require answers, who want to do the same thing over and over again: spirituality is for those who want to find new paths, do different things. And that is what supervision is about. Good supervisors live with the polarities:

- a definite way versus keeping it vague and open
- finding it myself versus inheriting it from others
- individual versus communal
- subjective versus objective
- one way (one truth) versus many ways (many truths).

In *Anam Cara*, a recent book on Celtic spirituality, the author, John O'Donohue (1997) has a very striking image of the human soul:

> It is helpful to visualise the mind as a tower of windows. Sadly, many people remain trapped at the one window, looking out every day at the same scene in the same way. Real growth is experienced when you draw back from that one window, turn and walk around the inner tower of the soul and see all the different windows that await your gaze. Through these different windows, you can see new vistas of possibility, presence and creativity. Complacency, habit and blindness often prevent you from feeling your life. So much depends on the frame of vision – the window through which we look. (p.163–4)

The spirituality of supervision is about being curious, fresh and ready for surprises. The qualifications for being a supervisor of surprises are:

- a teller of stories and jokes
- a giver of little gifts
- one who smiles and one who cries
- a dreamer
- one who surprises and is surprised
- one who has no avarice.

Spiritual people are feedback-people: feedback is received and given because in feedback we learn and grow. We welcome life-giving feedback from others that helps us grow and learn and remain forever young. For spirituality is about being young: there is no old age in spirituality. It's called wisdom and accompanies reflection and learning and little to do with chronological age. Supervisors are forever young: they intend playing more, creating more, stopping more, learning all the time. The life blood of supervision is learning as is playing (Hawkins and Shohet 1987), for it is in play that learning is at its highest: when there is relaxation, curiosity, wonder, challenge and creativity. Oscar Wilde challenges us: 'Only the shallow know themselves', he writes, 'if you know yourself you have not touched the depths'.

3. Becoming process oriented

For all of us there are depths, processes within, underlying issues that have remained untouched and unseen. There is more to each of us than what is visible. There are no quick fixes, for me, for you, for us. There is no path that is not emotional and painful. We have to break chains to be free and forge relationships to be connected. What was a freedom yesterday becomes all too easily a prison today and a death tomorrow. How can I trust myself and my own processes and those of others without being naive and gullible? Spirituality is about knowing my own processes and respecting the processes of others.

Sam Keen (1994) talks about 'constructing a spiritual bullshit detector'. I have adapted his idea to construct a 'supervisor bullshit detector', which comes in the form of 'Beware of ...' So, beware of ...

- charismatic supervisors, unquestioned authorities, enlightened masters, perfect gurus, reincarnated teachers and particularly supervisors who have discovered the only valid form of therapy. You will only end up seeing life and clients through their eyes and not your own. You will know this kind of supervisor because they will demand that you be like them
- supervisors who demand obedience: they have not discovered that there are other people in the world and want to keep you as a child
- supervisors who lead double lives. Look carefully at your supervisor's personal life: are there double standards, are they asking from you what they do not do themselves?
- supervisors who have only disciples. Check to see if your supervisor has friends, peer relationships and a community of equals, or only disciples
- supervisors who have achieved universal compassion but lack the capacity for simple friendships. Keep in mind what Dag Hammarskjold (1964) once said: 'It is more noble to give yourself completely to one individual than to labour diligently for the salvation of the masses.' (p.116)

- supervisors who do not encourage difference of opinion, challenge, criticism and discussion. Good supervisors are open to whatever truth comes knocking on the supervisory door
- supervisors who demand that you put loyalty to them above loyalty to friends or family, especially those who put down other supervisors and ask you to take sides
- supervisors who have no sense of humour. Test your supervisor to see how much humour and poking of fun about beliefs, slogans and dogmas is permissible. The absence of humour is an almost certain sign that you should pack your psychological bags and get the hell out of there. The first thing deadly serious fanatical rulers and organisations do is to forbid satire, repress the clowns, silence the jesters and kill levity.

Finally, before every supervision session check the batteries on your supervisor bullshit detector to make sure the detector is in good working order.

Trusting the process is at the heart of spirituality. The process is not to control but to allow to happen and to celebrate. We do what we can and we allow the process to take over. Then strange things happen: clients we have given up on change, a new trainee works miracles where old timers have failed, the impossible and the unthinkable begin to take place.

4. Establishing healthy relationships

The spirituality of supervision is about healthy and healing relationships. Carl Rogers (1980) was right – healthy relationships create healthy people. But healthy relationships need to be established and sustained and nurtured. Trying to care for our relationships and ourselves too often results in unbalance. Kottler (1986) writes of this imbalance:

> I have always found it ironic that clients who pay for my time, people whom I would rarely choose as friends, nevertheless receive 95 per cent of my attention, my focused concentration. Yet, the people I truly love the most get me in diluted form, distracted and self-involved. As I am writing these words my son calls my name. I put him off, 'Be with you in a minute. Let me finish what I am doing'. Now I would never do that with a client whose ramblings were interrupting an important thought. I give my best away to people who pay for my time. Must my son make an appointment to get my undivided attention.

The spirituality of supervision says look after your loved ones as you look after your clients, look after yourself as well as you look after your clients.

Good supervisors patrol the boundary walls of relationships to ensure that they remain healthy. They know how easy it is to become abusive, punitive, game-playing and hurtful (Page 1999). They know and practice the skill of how to be an individual and still not be ego-centred.

James Fowler and Sam Keen (1978) take a different stance towards developmental theory that might be more applicable to supervision and its values. They talk of five stages within this development:

> *Child*: Characterised by being with others but being dependent.
>
> *Rebel*: Against others (how can you be a saint if you have never been a sinner?).
>
> *Adult*: Co-operating with others.
>
> *Outlaw*: On being alone and being shocking.
>
> *Lover/fool*: Nevertheless … I trust.

Understanding these stages, through which both supervisor and supervisee travel, alone and together, in one-to-one relationships and groups, allows supervisors and supervisees to stay with each other and their processes. This is the spiritual journey as well as the supervisory one.

5. Learning connnectedness

Both spirituality and supervision look for connections. A few years ago a book entitled *The In-between God* was written by a theologian in which he argued that God existed between people, and he was at the in-between places. God, he surmised, connected people to people, culture to culture, people to environment and earth. Spirituality, like counselling and supervision, is about seeing, maintaining and holding connections. Martin Buber suggests we move to the 'sphere of the between', from which vantage point we can question the healthiness of any religion, any spirituality and any supervision that does not purport to be a 'bridge' to others.

Thorne (1997), who writes passionately of the need for the spiritual within the realm of counselling, speaks of this connection as at the heart of spirituality:

> It is because I am essentially a human being that I am, whether I know it or not or whether I like it or not, indisputably linked to all that has been or will be. I am not an isolated entity but rather a unique part of the whole created order. (p.206)

At the heart of spirituality is connectedness. We know we are related to one another, connected by human bonds. We know we are connected to the earth, to animals, to each other. We are not isolated and alone. Whether it is chaos theory that reminds us of these connections and patterns or systems theory that connects everything, deep within is a tie we cannot break. Keen (1994) considers system theory as the modern glue that binds many sciences together:

> Systems theory has emerged as the dominant trend in most disciplines, from psychology to computer science, replacing the old method of piecemeal analysis, in which we broke everything down into its component parts. The tendency in recent thought is to stress synthesis, networks, interaction, and process. The old notion that the whole is the sum of the parts has been replaced by the idea that the parts can only be understood as functions of the dynamics of the whole. The 19th Century vision of lonely billiard-ball atoms accidentally colliding with each other to form the varieties of life has been replaced by a vision of a universe made up of an intricate web of relationships, a net of jewels. (p.xxi)

Connectedness is about going beyond. I am, after all, not the centre of the universe, a humbling stance that allows me to let go and allow others to connect to me in appropriate ways. Supervision is about making such connections – in some, strange, mysterious, convoluted, interesting, unsuspecting way, it's all connected.

6. Becoming an interior person

Someone once said that when you stand before yourself you stand before God. We are interior people who go inside to find ourselves and indeed others. But it not easy: 'The longest journey is the journey inwards' (Hammarskjold 1964, p.65). A basic principle of spirituality is that we should trust our deepest desires, and our values tell us about who we are and what we are: 'If we become addicted to the external our interiority will haunt us.' (O'Donohue 1997, p.14.)

We go within to find the principles that guide us. What are the principles for the spirituality of supervision? Frank Koch in *Proceedings*, the magazine of the Naval Institute, tells the story of the need for principles:

> Two battleships assigned to the training squadron had been at sea on manoeuvres in heavy weather for several days. I was serving on the lead battleship and was on watch on the bridge as night fell. The visibility was poor with patchy fog, so the captain remained on the bridge keeping an eye on all activities. Shortly after dawn, the lookout on the wing of the bridge reported, 'Light, bearing on the starboard bow'. 'Is it steady or moving astern?' the captain called out. Lookout replied, 'Steady Captain', which meant we were on a dangerous collision course with that ship. The captain then called to the signalman 'Signal that ship: We are on a collision course, advise you change course 20 degrees'. Back came the signal, 'Advisable for you to change course 20 degrees'. The captain said, 'Send, I am a captain, change your course 20 degrees'. 'I'm a seaman second-class', came the reply, 'You had better change course 20 degrees'. By this time the captain was furious. He spat out, 'Send, I'm a battleship, Change your course 20 degrees.' Back came the flashing light, 'I'm a lighthouse'. We changed course. (Recounted in Covey 1989, p.33)

Principles are like lighthouses: they give us bearings. What are the principles of both spirituality and supervision?:

- fairness (equity and justice): no social or psychological exclusions
- integrity and honesty which create trust
- human dignity for all people
- service (making a contribution)
- excellence (without perfectionism)
- potential (we have enormous powers of growth)
- apologies, if and when needed.

Spirituality is about realism, it is about letting go in order to live. There is an old saying from medieval times that can still be a contemporary guide about living life: 'The monk', it says, 'begins to live the morning he wakes up and realises he'll never be a saint or never be abbot.' Prather (1972) puts it well too:

> If I had only ...
>
> forgotten future greatness
>
> and looked at the green things and the buildings
>
> and reached out to those around me
>
> and smelled the air
>
> and ignored the forms and the self-styled obligations
>
> and heard the rain on the roof
>
> and put my arms around my wife
>
> ... and it is not too late.

Supervision is a form of retreat: leaving our professional world, leaving our work for a while, we come to 'stop and listen' as the contemplative monk Thomas Merton is reputed to have replied when asked to define spirituality. Stopping and listening is the greatest spiritual act of all: listening to me, to my clients, to my supervisees, to my supervisors, to the organisation. We retreat in order to return different and, of course, when we are different so are others. Changes in me herald changes in others, changes in others herald changes in me. We are on a constant intermingling and interconnected pilgrimage, a journey to sacred places, not because the place of itself may be necessarily important but because pilgrimages are always about finding oneself, not inevitably getting to the destination.

The message and lesson at the heart of spirituality, and of supervision, is simple: 'In the last analysis you cannot be someone else, you only live and are and relate with the fullness of your humanity, not by conforming, but by becoming you. Go rummage around within.'

Conclusion

In summary, the spirituality of supervision is about having a cat asleep in your arms: 'I'm holding this cat in my arms so it can sleep, and what more is there' (Prather 1972). At that moment you can do nothing else, you are absolved from doing anything else. It should be declared unprofessional, unethical and probably illegal to do anything that might disturb the cat. How can you do anything else – when there is a cat asleep in your lap, that is the end of the story. Cat-lovers know this. Others, unfortunately, don't and disturb what should not be disturbed.

Spirituality and supervision are about shifts in mentality from:

- the unexamined life to continual reflection
- the same things over and over again to new ways
- individual to communal
- isolation to connectedness
- exterior to interior
- sameness to surprises
- static to developmental
- head to head and heart
- competition to co-operation
- greed to generosity
- denial to facing monsters.

Maybe the word 'movement' gives the wrong impression. Perhaps the whole exercise is about integrating these opposites into a unified whole. R. D. Laing should have the last word, which is probably the best spiritual and supervisory principle of all: 'There is nothing to be afraid of.'

References

Carroll, M. (2000) 'Learning, unlearning, relearning and not learning.' Private paper.

Covey, S. (1989) *The Seven Habits of Highly Effective People.* London: Simon and Schuster.

Fowler, J. and Keen, S. (1978) *Life Maps.* Waco, TX: World Books.

Hammarskjold, D. (1964) *Markings.* London: Faber and Faber.

Hawkins, P. and Shohet, R. (1987) *Supervision in the Helping Professions.* Buckinghamshire: Open University Press.

Keen, S. (1994) *Hymns to an Unknown God.* London: Piatkus.

Kottler, J. (1986) *On Being a Therapist.* San Francisco, CA: Jossey-Bass.

Neufeldt, S. (1999) 'Training in reflective processes in supervision.' In E. Holloway and M. Carroll (eds) *Training Counselling Supervisors: Strategies, Methods and Techniques.* London: Sage.

O'Donohue, J. (1997) *Anan Cara: Spiritual Wisdom from the Celtic World.* London: Bantam Press.

Page, S. (1999) *The Shadow and the Counsellor.* London: Routledge.

Prather, H. (1972) *Notes to Myself: My Struggle to Become a Person.* London: Lyrebird Press.

Rogers, C. (1980) *A Way of Being.* Boston, MA: Houghton Mifflin Company.

Thorne, B. (1997) 'Spiritual responsibility in a secular profession.' In I. Horton and V. Varma (eds) *The Needs of Counsellors and Psychotherapists.* London: Sage.

Thorne, B. (1998) 'Values and spirituality at work.' *Counselling at Work 21,* 3–4.

West, W. (2000) *Psychotherapy and Spirituality.* London: Sage.

PART 2

Supervision in Clinical Areas

Chapter 7

Supervision and the Mental Health of the Counsellor

Penny Henderson

Introduction

Supervision can have an impact on the work of counsellors in relation to their health. Age, stage of professional life, stage in the family life cycle, mental health and physical health all contribute to, or indeed take away from, the energy and resilience counsellors have available for counselling.

Middle-aged women make up the huge majority of counsellors and supervisors. I am a woman in my fifties, supervising many very experienced and competent women counsellors in their fifties. There seem to be a number of personal/professional dilemmas which are common to this age and stage of professional experience which affect supervision in significant ways. Some of these include the balance of time we spend on personal issues, the nature of the supervisory relationship and the focus on restorative functions. Later, the particular challenges of going through a similar life phase as my supervisees will be explored with particular emphasis on the benefits and drawbacks of this similarity for effective supervision.

My particular supervisory focus about health revolves around what has been called the normative and the restorative functions of supervision (Proctor and Inskipp 1993; 1995) as well as on the crucial importance for the supervisory relationship of regular reviews. By 'normative' is meant the ethical, administrative and professional aspects of the work and by 'restorative', the supportive containment of the supervisees' emotional experiences relating to the work.

I know about vulnerability, of course, from two positions, and want to talk about it from both. As a supervisor I have observed swings in supervisees' self-confidence, resilience, optimism and locus of control, and the impact of these on the quality and quantity of the work they do. I have sought to be a robust ally to help and support them to keep working and living well. As a counsellor I have received much steadying, comforting, clarifying, personal and professional help from my various supervisors at the times of my own personal vulnerability.

What is relevant and important in terms of the mental health of a counsellor as it is expressed in the supervisory relationships?

Attending to the mental health of the counsellor

The mental health of the counsellor can be ascertained by attending to:

- her capacity for empathy – can she put herself imaginatively and accurately into the client's world?
- her coherence of narrative – if incoherent she might be smiling while talking about painful matters, for example
- her agency – is she able to initiate, respond and undertake tasks she aims to do?
- her creativity – is she creative in her work and in relation to the supervisor in supervision?
- her self-awareness – can she tolerate her full range of emotions?

Some questions supervisors ask about the counsellor:

- is she open to new learning, and non-defensive in exploration of her work?
- is she able to give an account of the work which identifies her own part in it?
- is she able to express hurt and anger, sadness, delight, triumph and disappointment? How solid is her self-esteem? When is it wobbly?
- is she able to meet her own needs – at least some of the time even at the expense of others?
- is she is able to be disappointing sometimes, and to set boundaries and keep them? Is she able to ask for care in reciprocal relationships, and when appropriate, in supervision? Most particularly, is she able to be congruent in her relationships with her clients, herself and with me?
- is she vulnerable or fierce, responsive or uncomfortable in relation to me as her supervisor? If she is open, and issues are acknowledged, then they can be worked on.

In contrast, the possibility of mental ill health in the counsellor is relevant to the supervisor, largely in the converse of the list just outlined. One extreme is when the supervisee is dismissive of her clients and shows no inclination to explore why she is unable to help them. She locates the problems in the clients who are said to be uncommitted, unreliable, resistant, or who have 'probably done enough' even when they leave prematurely and without saying goodbye. When the counsellor is rigid, preoccupied with self, judgmental or apparently totally out of touch with her client's reality then the supervisor is right to be worried.

One supervisee was quick to anger, opinionated, very resistant to personal explorations in relation to her work with her clients, and with very strong views which affected her approach to clients. She seemed very vulnerable and needy, yet unable to ask for or receive care from the supervisor who felt she had to 'tread on eggshells' with the supervisee, rather than respond freely offering a mix of support and challenge. She, the supervisee, had been counselling in a voluntary organisation for a couple of years and had had three previous supervisors because of changes in staffing, so her present supervisor felt she was entitled to some anger. But when the supervisor did, belatedly, attend to her growing concern, and raise the courage to explore these worries they rapidly got stuck in an impasse of 'I do my best' versus 'We must be able to talk about what *you* are doing in the counselling relationship'. The supervisee would neither accept a 'restorative' focus, nor engage with a 'normative' exchange. The supervisor insisted the voluntary organisation talk with her about these issues, and ceased to supervise her.

Good learning from this experience for the supervisor was to attend to the countertransference responses as in the tentative 'treading on eggshells' above, attending to the extreme sleepiness, or unusual boredom within herself during supervision and to use them to explore with the supervisee whether the supervisory relationship is serving her needs, the supervisor's and the needs of the clients. The supervisor records her responses in supervisory notes so that the patterns of them can be monitored and explored in her own supervision.

Relevant issues about mental ill health seem very often to be expressed physically too: frequent susceptibility to colds, sore throats or 'flu, bad backs, migraine and exhaustion, especially when it occurs at approximately the same time each year, is relevant. It usually affects the resilience and optimism of the counsellor and triggers the supervisor to suggest a 'normative' review about workloads and energy levels.

Bright spots and other distortions

It is interesting to speculate how far age, gender and cultural background affect what Eckstein (1969) calls the counsellor's or supervisor's blind spots, dumb spots and deaf spots. He defines the dumb spots as matters about which the counsellor is ignorant; blind spots are her own personal patterns and prejudices which get in the way of seeing the client clearly; and deaf spots are those defensive reactions which prevent her from hearing the client or the supervisor. Burton (personal communication) adds 'bright spots', that is, those strong interests of the counsellor or supervisor which pull her to focus on matters of existing interest or concern to her.

All my supervisees at one point or another have felt very depleted and exhausted, and begun to long for their next break. (This may also be true of 100 per cent of the rest of the adult population and most school children in the UK today as well!). I am aware how many times that supervisees mention low mood, exhaustion, their own ill health, or a deeply debilitating overload arising from other roles such as family carers in addition to their work.

Examples from my own supervisory work include:

- in the last nine years, my 17 supervisees have between them had ten bereavements of close kin, and two are active carers of parents with Alzheimer's
- seven have had to miss supervision or counselling sessions because of their own illnesses, exhaustion, operations or accidents
- during this period, I think that 9 out of 17 supervisees have experienced episodes of mild to moderate depression. In almost every depression the trigger has been a life event related to ill-health or loss, to work overload, or to an anniversary reaction to a bereavement.

Approximately ten per cent of the general population experiences depression. There is no evidence about how many counsellors or supervisors experience depression but it could be assumed that a similar, or perhaps even a greater, proportion do.

There is considerable and useful writing about the training of counsellors and the impact of the demands of the training experience on the resilience of trainees in this time of transition and growth. Trainers do have some responsibility to monitor and consider (and also assess) the mental health of trainees. Personal development does not stop when training ends: restorative supervision provides an ongoing space and relationship for exploration and sharing in service of personal development.

Sometimes a shared experience can be very moving as in the following example. One counsellor was reporting on work with a client whose baby had died when she was one week old and recently the client's 24-year-old son had been killed in an accident. The counsellor talked to me of her own baby who had died when six hours old and she wept as she spoke of her memories of returning to the grave 17 years later. Tears came to my eyes, and I then told her about the baby I had had who died at seven months old and had no grave but had been given to medical research. She and I both now have healthy living sons. For a moment we shared tears about the pain of loving children who die and fears for those who live. Then we returned to focus on her work with her client with a more heartfelt compassion from our sharing, and a deeper sense of connection between ourselves knowing we understood a little bit more about each other.

There are three possibilities of supervisory focus which need particular attention in relation to sustaining the mental health of the counsellor. They are:

1. Reviewing the counsellor's motivation to be a counsellor.
2. Monitoring her resilience with the counsellor, and how it affects her attitude to clients and to her practice.
3. Talking about self-care.

1. Reviewing the counsellor's motivation to be a counsellor

Two basic questions to identify counsellor motivation may be 'What made you decide you want to be a counsellor?' and 'What are you getting out of it these days?' The BAC code of ethics (1998) for counsellors states that: 'Counsellors are responsible for ensuring that their relationships with clients are not unduly influenced by their own emotional needs.' Many counsellors are aware of the role their own needs play: to be liked, to soothe their own hurts projectively, to be loveable, to be worthy, to meet their own intimacy needs, or needs to be helpful, to be thanked and to build their own self-esteem by doing a good job. When the work is not going well supervisees may report feeling burdened by the neediness of their clients, and unable to protect themselves from the pain or the stuckness. Then it is important to reflect on the part their own needs are playing in creating this response to their counselling work.

2. Monitoring the counsellor's resilience, and how it affects her attitude to clients and to her practice

This task relates to the clause B1.12 in the BAC (1996) code of ethics for supervisors which states that:

> Supervisors are responsible for helping their supervisees recognise when their functioning as counsellors is impaired due to personal or emotional difficulties, any condition which affects judgement, illness, the influence of alcohol or drugs or for any other reason, and for ensuring that appropriate action is taken.

Appropriate action may take the form of a discussion with the supervisee about workload management, explorations about remaining reliable when suffering from an intermittent illness or about the challenges of being reliable when caught up with the needs of their own dependants. Explorations may be about ethical issues arising from having too many caring roles at home as well as at work and how to rest and recover, or stop, when she is also feeling responsible for seeing clients who are not at a suitable point for a break and whom she thinks need continuing weekly counselling.

Can one 'do good while feeling bad'? Manning (1995) writes of her own serious depression while working as a psychotherapist. On one occasion when she was going through the DSM IV list of nine factors predicting depression with a client she found she qualified for all nine when the client only rated five: 'The rapport between us feels solid and workable. But I wonder to myself how someone who is nine for nine on the depression index can possibly help someone who is only five for nine.' (p.76)

'Feeling bad' physically or psychologically will affect how counsellors engage with clients and can also be a reaction to how clients 'are' with the counsellor. If the counsellor knows that her own tears or fears, frustration or despair are near the surface she needs to keep them accessible and release them outside the counselling session, perhaps through singing, dancing, artwork, music making or meditation, sport or the comfort of intimates. Supervision is also a place where these feelings can be expressed and held.

Of course, there needs to be a clear contract between supervisor and supervisee that supervision is not primarily or frequently a therapy space. The focus on supervisory exploration about this person and her counselling work cannot be lost, even for those who do not have their own therapy and need therapeutic help at the time. Instead, a learning focus can allow exploration of how the counsellor is looking after herself, and how she can enable herself to keep on learning in the interests of her own development and the work with the clients. This includes learning to sustain her own well-being in hard times which is essential for the work and important for modelling to clients. Like the 'hidden curriculum' in schools, how we are and what our behaviour implies is part of what the client sees. The supervisor too needs to reflect about what she is modelling to her supervisees.

Carroll's clear discussion (1996) of the *counselling task* of the supervisor focuses on the supervision about the reactions of the counsellor to their work with clients. An additional focus is on workload management, caseload management and the resilience of the counsellor to meet the commitments she has made.

As Bolen (1994) argues about depression and the 'dark night of the soul', to work without any sense of play is depleting. Unless souls are nourished, she argues, men and women who work just for duty or the pay cheque often find themselves suffering from mid-life depressions. She relates the mid-life crisis to the sacrifice of the animus in work and suggests that depression which is masked as illness creates work characterised by lack of creativity. Supervisors have a responsibility, shared with the supervisee, to identify staleness or dutifulness in counselling work, and to stay creative themselves.

3. Talking about self-care

The BAC code of ethics for supervisors (clause B3.3.2) states that

> If, in the course of counselling supervision, it appears that personal counselling may be necessary for the supervisee to be able to continue to work effectively, the supervisor should raise this issue with the supervisee (1996).

When depletion affects personal self-acceptance, self-actualisation, the capacity for autonomy or the use of talents, it needs to be addressed. When the counsellor feels out of control and unable to comfort herself or accept comfort, therapy needs to be recommended as an option. For those supervisees who carry too many clients, or who cannot say no to requests for extra sessions, the chilling image of the frog who was put into a pot of water while the temperature was raised by slow degrees comes to mind. Unaware of the increasing heat and pressure, it allowed itself to be boiled without jumping out of the pot. At which degree of stress, distress, low spirit or preoccupation does the conscientious counsellor or supervisor 'jump out of the pot' and take time off? How often does the supervisor invite the counsellor to review the pot of water she is in and make plans for change that are realistic? How many get sick, or die, because they will not do so?

It is the combination of difficulties which some of the women in the fifties age group have faced which make these questions particularly pertinent. Seligman, in writing about learned helplessness (1975) and learned optimism (1991) reminds us that our explanatory styles affect whether we collapse under pressure or look for options. He notes three elements, which differ between the optimists and the pessimists:

1. Our view of what it is in our power to change (our locus of control).
2. Our view of the permanence of the difficulty.
3. Our belief of the pervasiveness of the difficulty.

Chronic illness can feel permanent, pervasive and out of control in a very debilitating way for the counsellor herself, or for her in her role as a carer.

The same-age supervisor's responses to the counsellor enmeshed in these webs of relationship may spring from the compassion of being on a very parallel journey and result in countertransferential reactions. It is essential to take time to explore the restorative issues, and if need be, to take the opportunity to exercise some supervisory authority. The responsibility of the practitioner to herself is to sustain the best mental and physical health she can in the circumstances, and that of the supervisor is to comment when that is palpably being undermined by workload or inner injunctions. It depends on the counsellor's awareness and readiness to address her own issues whether or not the supervisor intervenes. It may even entail the supervisor drawing the issues *insistently* to the counsellor's attention. It is hard to judge how bad it has to get before the supervisor also insists on actions such as reduction of caseload or stopping work. In the end, I have refused to continue to supervise one accredited counsellor whose lack of self-care, in my view, was a danger to her clients in a period of illness. She would not take time off.

The BAC code of ethics sets out the self-care principles for counsellors. This task relates to the clause B1.12 code of ethics for supervisors (1996) which I've mentioned, and it applies similarly for supervisors too. In section B 2.5 it states that

> Supervisors are responsible for withdrawing from counselling and supervision work either temporarily or permanently when their functioning is impaired due to personal or emotional difficulties, illness, the influence of alcohol, or drugs, or for any other reason.

While committed in principle to this code we cannot pretend that it is easy to apply. Counsellors also have loyalties to clients, ex-clients who wish to return, colleagues and employers, as well as individual personal pressures from mortgages, rent, credit cards or debts. It is a problematic tightrope to walk, hence the importance of having permission to take care of oneself. Like the counsellors, I, too, have heard myself say: 'When I am with the clients I am able to focus, it's only afterwards I realise how totally exhausted I am.' In these instances, if the supervisor is not modelling limit setting, who brings this to the attention of the counsellor–supervisor dyad? This is where peer supervision, especially in a group, can provide a useful opportunity, and this may be a distinct function which it is worth contracting to monitor.

How many counsellors or supervisors can say, hand on heart, that they have not worked while their functioning is impaired? One question is *how much* does it need to be impaired before it is essential to cease work? Another is *what sorts of* impairment is it most necessary to monitor: exhaustion? poor memory? concentration? depression? capacity to make psychological contact? resilience? something else? If the supervisor is in the same life stage as the counsellor, is she generally better placed or not to recognise, explore, and if necessary confront this?

Maintaining good mental health for the caring professional

Suggestions for maintaining good mental health for supervisees include at least six supervisory interventions, all of which I have found helpful to use myself and to tell others over the years.

1. To have regular reviews which take stock and clarify the counsellor's motivation to do the work and the satisfactions and costs of doing it. If the counsellor is 'living with zest in an empty nest' by becoming

'Mother Hubbard' to others, the power imbalances or co-dependency issues may usefully be explored. For example, children of alcoholics are at risk of becoming 'overfunctioners' addicted to helping in order to be in control.

2. To explore whether the counsellor has reciprocal relationships amongst friends and family to counterbalance the essentially dependent ones with clients. Is this just a sub-cultural norm, or is it professionally important that the counsellor allows herself to receive as well as to give? If because of geographical moves or family losses there are no significant reciprocal relationships, should I, as I do as a supervisor, encourage the counsellor to review her support arrangements, and if need be pay for her own therapy, massage and so forth? This deals with the issue of support but not with the inability to choose and sustain relationships characterised by reciprocity. I expect all my supervisees to have had some therapy to meet BAC guidelines, and to seek out more if they need it. I do believe this is good practice on many levels for any counsellor, but I do not insist that they are currently in therapy.

3. To discuss what else sustains supervisees' emotional resilience – to avoid the Scylla of burnout or the Charybdis of a cynical hardening of the heart. Getting a good balance of work and play, excitation and relaxation, exercise and stillness, and warm human interaction outside the counselling and supervision rooms is essential to good work as a counsellor.

4. To invite counsellors to develop what I have come to call 'the Velcro solution'. That is, view layers of emotional protection like an onion, and encourage counsellors to learn to add or remove them appropriately; removing them to be free to be close to friends and family; and to be empathic with clients, and walk accurately in their worlds, but replacing them with more disturbing people, or colleagues or others who require an assertive and determined form of interaction. Broom (1997) writes about 'intimacy skills "necessary for doctors"' and describes self-awareness, respect, assertiveness, 'a willingness to "go near the edge" in a relationship' (pp.62–63) and links these with willingness to confront. It can be liberating to counsellor and supervisor alike to accept that anyone is free to take an unhealthy course if they so choose. Some student doctors are now also taught 'de-empathising skills' so they can move on and engage with the next patient in a busy surgery. How many counselling or supervision courses address this issue? Should supervisors do so?

5. To identify boundaries and focus, limits and priorities. This may mean identifying what supervisees will stop doing whatever the incentives are to continue. These may include that she is good at it, or she likes doing it, or she is fond of the people she does it with. But in order to focus, and keep work within limits which are manageable to the available energy of this life stage, she may benefit if she reduces or eliminates particular chunks of work. In the words of Estes (1992, p.317) it means being willing to be ruthless enough about one's own creative or restorative activities to have an actual or metaphorical notice on the door which says: 'I am working (or resting) here today and I am not receiving visitors. I know you do not think this is you because you are my banker, agent or best friend. But it does.' To have the strength of will not to answer the phone or door or check the emails will always take an effort. Some people, peers inform me, have permission to monitor their own energy levels and can avoid answering the door or the phone effortlessly. I find this potentially admirable and amazing.
6. To consider how far lifestyle and level of well-being can be a model to clients. So many of us bargain with our bodies, to last out until the next break. Some re-framing is necessary, which is not to identify the 'I' with willpower, not to live the mind–body split – but to entitle the self to a well-balanced life with the power of the will exercised on behalf of the body. Much easier said than done, says this tepid, and sometimes hot, frog.

Reviews

Regular reviews between supervisor and counsellor are essential, and the work I have done to write this chapter has been immensely productive in highlighting themes and patterns in the supervisory relationships I have reviewed. The initial contract-making discussion often introduces the key themes. At intervals, supervisor and supervisee can usefully reflect on what the counsellor has got or not got from supervision in the period reviewed; what targets to set for the next period; new learning, a focus for reflection, what to audit and what the supervisor needs to change.

As supervisor I seem constantly to be inviting supervisees to review their workloads: 'Is 180 clients in individual and group therapy too many? How would you know?'; 'Is work in three GP practices at the same time too much?' (Mentioning that up to 18,000 people could, in theory, call on her services made this question real). Reviews are so useful, especially just before or just after a holiday or break, when the impact of the work on the energy level of the counsellor is most vivid. I know there is a shift downhill when my supervisees or I come less prepared for supervision. The opposite is signalled when we have had time and spare energy to prepare and to undertake reviews of their work.

Sometimes the counsellor becomes aware of the supervisor's low energy or burnout, and the question arises 'Can she do or say something about this? Is this relationship robust and open enough for the observations to be mentioned and explored?' What the supervisor models to the counsellor can and should be named. For example. one young volunteer counsellor who is very intuitive said to me that she had gone away from our previous session of supervision, aware that I was 'not OK' but neither of us had commented about it. She had felt it was her fault and it really knocked her self-confidence about counselling. I had unintentionally been sound asleep when she arrived, after a particularly powerful therapy session for myself, and I hadn't acknowledged this. Her initiative allowed us to clear it up.

Another experienced counsellor whom I had supervised for five years announced she had found another supervisor. She said I'd sowed the seeds the previous year in a review by asking her to identify when she would know it would be the right time to change supervisors. She began the next, our last, session with 'I felt I'd hurt you last time', and thus took the initiative to explore the mix of feelings we both had. I had been surprised, had felt the loss and didn't express it immediately as I digested her news, partly because I assumed she had decided to leave because I had been ill the previous summer. Actually she had attended a training with someone and wanted to try supervision with her. Her intervention allowed me to check for the grain of truth in my paranoia that my being ill, and therefore unreliable, in that time was the central reason for her decision. My own 'be perfect' driver had stopped me commenting at the time.

The menopause: an example of a life stage issue

When the counsellor's energy is low or unreliable or her memory is impaired by depression or menopause, it requires a huge effort to marshal resources in service of the work. Chronic physical or mental illness in herself or close kin is in actuality a matter which takes great organisation to respond to while working reliably. Many of the women in my small sample negotiated this physical and psychological transition with difficulty. For some, that included what were potentially life-threatening experiences which not only undermined well-being and energy levels, but also affected the capacity to be reliably available for the clients. This is an age when women are more susceptible to the various chronic ailments associated with the later part of life, and to the lower energy levels associated with the menopausal period.

Ruderman (in Cantor 1990), studying the countertransference themes of women therapists working with women clients, writes, 'Most striking was the profound resonance, going beyond empathy, that the therapists experience, especially around issues of mid-life, menopause and pre menopause' (p.14). And Levy adds to this (Cantor 1990):

> Long-standing female identification processes rooted in the early mother/daughter relationship produce a situation where both female therapists and their female clients will most likely struggle with intense issues around identification and nurturance. (p.14)

Sheehy (1993) reminds us that hot flushes and flooding are both quintessentially about being out of control, which for some women connects to depression. She alerts readers to cultural, dietary and exercise differences across cultures which lead some women in particular countries, including our own, not to report difficulties in this period. She encourages women to 'claim the pause' and asserts that those who master the art of letting go gracefully, who address fears of ageing and death in their fifties, may come through to fine-tuned priorities and focus and post-menopausal zest, with a capacity for vitality lasting into their eighties and nineties. Though there may be less vitality, resilience or immunity to depression in this time, these may go hand in hand with a necessary and exciting learning to prioritise her own needs more, the development of acceptance of who she is and an increase in her own capacity to set limits and boundaries and exercise power and influence. It is not by any means all a story of diminution. Yet the supervisee, who is going through a difficult time, can be immensely reassured to have a known and trusted supervisor who remembers her in less vulnerable times, and reminds her of her competence even if she has temporarily 'forgotten what it is like to feel well' and thus lacks confidence.

Profound resonance or struggles with issues around identification and nurturance seem liable to affect these supervisory relationships too. A consequence can be a wish to support the supervisee through a series of crises (I would not like to be the sort of supervisor who does not do this). Yet this also must be balanced by the longer term expectation of a professional level of preparation for supervision and regular reviews of the caseload or enough focus on the clients. Without regular reviews it is easier to fail to undertake the normative functions of supervision. Clearly the challenge to the female supervisor, like the female therapist, is to notice and explore these issues and countertransferences.

There can also be dissonance, for example, the 'wise woman' supervisor who is also vulnerable. When relevant because of supervisees' patterns, life style and difficulties with workload management, I share with them that I struggle with workaholism, saying no and taking good enough care of myself. It has taken me years to do this as well as I do now. I wonder when is this a useful bit of modelling, as a wounded healer struggling honestly with similar issues, and how this shared world can pull one to collude in ways that a supervisor of a different age or gender or orientation would not? I think it makes me more aware of the internal dynamics, in the 'set a thief to catch a thief' mode, and it highlights the importance of having supervision about supervision.

If the supervisor is in the midst of experiencing similar life events to her supervisees, she must be particularly aware of and control her bright spot urges about it, as she must monitor any urge to take undue control. Yet, here may also be a powerful point of honest connection, which may be healing to both hearts, a moment of meeting where reciprocity is more useful than distance. What I've become aware of is a variety of changes in the relationship as supervisees see me as more vulnerable. Some really like it, and feel much freer to be themselves, 'warts and all'. Others respond (for example, to an operation) by bringing cards, gifts or flowers, and this can be extremely welcome in a hard time. There is also a question do such gifts alter the supervisory relationship, and if so, how? Has anyone thought about the meaning of gifts in supervision, and the timing of them at Christmas or in response to special events? Some respond by 'not being too heavy', for example one supervisee suggested we stop a session early because she thought I looked too tired. Some, by enquiring, reduce a previous distance as they know more about me personally, and the state of my health. This can be useful in reducing any idealisations still left after years of a shared supervisory relationship, but could also limit the usefulness of supervision if the supervisee takes on an inappropriately mothering role. It is not what they are paying for. And it may seem very ungrateful, though necessary, to ask if the supervisee may be inappropriately mothering her clients in a similar way.

Certainly the relationship needs to be robust enough for the supervisee to express her reactions to being 'let down', and any fears such as 'breaks in the frame' create about survival and well-being in someone on whom she may depend to some degree. If she herself is also vulnerable and struggling with parallel issues it may be hard for a supervisee to initiate such exchanges, as whatever she may say to her supervisor may also apply to her as a counsellor from the client's perspective.

I can recall no writing that explores reactions in supervision to the vulnerability of a male supervisor who is facing mid-life issues, bereavement, chronic illness or family crises. Does this indicate that expectations of women supervisors are different? Would a male or a female supervisee expect to take flowers or a gift to a male supervisor in these circumstances? Some do, I am told, but if not, why not? Would they expect to respond to him by not being 'too heavy', or ask questions about his condition and how he is coping? And whatever the answers, the interesting question is 'How does this change in the relationship affect the way supervisor and supervisee work in the interests of the development of the supervisee and the safety of the clients?'

Conclusion

In conclusion, some of the questions which I think may be useful to counsellors and their supervisors are:

- what are we doing in supervision to help improve the quality of psychological contact you have with your clients?
- are we usefully uncomfortable enough, or are we being collusive?
- how would you notice whether you need to go back into therapy? If your own current issues affect your relationship with your clients or your own well-being, should you return to therapy?
- what am I modelling to you in my behaviour as your supervisor? What are you (and I) teaching by example? Are we satisfied with this? How does it help your clients?
- is my supervisory voice in your head an encouraging or an inhibiting one? How good am I at offering an alternative view without undermining the supervisory relationship or your self-confidence?
- what evidence do we have of the effectiveness of our supervision?

As we emphasise this effectiveness, I think that we need to keep squarely in our sights the emotional containment which supports the mental *health* of the counsellor, and thus her capacity to reflect creatively on her work with her clients.

Acknowledgements and appreciation

First to my supervisees who have taught me so much. Second, to colleagues and friends with whom I have discussed the ideas in this chapter. You know who you are. Thank you.

References

British Association for Counselling (1996) *Code of Ethics and Practice for Supervisors.* Rugby: BAC.

British Association for Counselling (1998) *Code of Ethics and Practice for Counsellors.* Rugby: BAC.

Bolen, J. S. (1994) *Crossing to Avalon – A woman's mid-life Pilgrimage.* San Francisco, CA: Harper.

Broom, B. (1997) *Somatic Illness and the Patient's Other Story.* London: Free Association Books.

Cantor, D. W. (1990) (ed) *Women as Therapists.* London: Jason Aronson.

Carroll, M. (1996) *Counselling Supervision.* London: Cassell.

Eckstein, R. (1969) 'Concerning the teaching and learning of psychoanalysis.' *Journal of the American Psychoanalytical Association 17*, 2, 312–332.

Estes, C. P. (1992) *Women who Run with the Wolves.* London: Random House.

Levy, S. B. (1982) 'Towards a consideration of intimacy in the female/female therapist relationship.' *Women and Therapy 1*, 2, 35–44.

Manning, M. (1995) *Undercurrents: A Therapist's Reckoning with Depression.* San Francisco, CA: Harper.

Proctor, B. and Inskipp, F. (1993) *The Art, Craft, and Tasks of Counselling Supervision Part 1 'Making the most of supervision'.* Twickenham: Cascade.

Proctor' B. and Inskipp, F. (1995) *The Art, Craft and Tasks of Counselling Supervision Part 2 'Becoming a supervisor',* Twickenham: Cascade

Seligman, M. (1975) *Helplessness: On Depression, Development and Death.* New York: Freeman Press.

Seligman, M. (1991) *Learned Optimism.* New York: Random House.

Sheehy, G. (1993) *The Silent Passage.* London: Harper Collins.

Further reading

Dass, R. and Gorman, P. (1985) *How can I help?* San Francisco, CA: Rider.

Grosch, W. N. and Olsen, D. C. (1994) *When Helping starts to Hurt: A New Look at Burnout Among Psychotherapists.* New York: W. W. Norton.

Guggenbuhl-Craig, A. (1971) *Power in the Helping Professions.* TX: Spring Publications.

Hawkins, P. and Shohet, R. (1989) *Supervision in the Helping Professions.* Milton Keynes: OU Press.

Ruderman, E. G. (1986) 'Gender related themes of women psychotherapists in their treatment of women patients: the creative and reparative use of counter transference as a mutual growth experience.' *Clinical Social Work Journal 14*, 2, 103–126.

Skovholt, T.M. and Rønnestad, M.H. (1995) *The Evolving Professional Self.* Chichester: Wiley.

Chapter 8

Counselling Supervision in Primary Health Care

Graham Curtis Jenkins

Introduction

Over the past 20 years, counsellors and psychotherapists increasingly have found work in primary health care, initially using what was, in effect, a private practice model of service delivery. In late 1998, the first National Survey of Counsellors working in UK general practices revealed that counsellors were working in more than half of all UK general practices (Mellor-Clarke, Simms Ellis and Burton 2001). Over time therapists of all persuasions and backgrounds have struggled to develop efficient, effective, respectful service models to meet the needs of patients who were no longer called clients. The general practice in which they worked and the needs of the wider local community including other health service environments like mental health services have helped mould the model (Curtis Jenkins 1999).

The survey also revealed, for the first time, exactly how ingenious and creative counsellors were in delivering brief therapy services in general practice. The counsellors had found out for themselves (and with the aid of a tiny number of dedicated training providers) how to deliver a totally new way of working, blending therapy approaches, matching the approach to the patient – and not vice versa as is commonly believed (and perhaps less often practised by 'single model' therapists). The national survey showed that counsellors were using a range of therapy modalities including Gestalt, cognitive behavioural, integrative as well as solution focused therapy approaches in addition to their person centred or psychodynamic core models.

Effectiveness of counselling in primary care

More and more randomised control trials of brief therapy interventions by counsellors in naturalistic settings show that the therapists are undertaking the skilful task of effective 'jobbing psychotherapy'. We know that these counsellors are effective at enabling important psychotherapeutic gains to be made, remoralising patients, remediating them and very rarely rehabilitating them (Howard, Orlinsky and Jueger 1999), such therapists having given up the concept of cure as a goal of therapy. We now know for instance that this 'brief' therapy delivered by counsellors for patients with depression and anxiety is probably more effective for patients with depression than cognitive behaviour therapy in primary health care settings. We also know that a majority of patients maintain their improvement at two year follow up and the more depressed the patient was at initial assessment, the more likely they are to stay well (Baker *et al.* 1998).

Equally interesting is that other important effects of these primary care psychological therapy services are beginning to emerge. Many studies have now shown that once a patient has seen a counsellor they tend to see their GP less. As patients seen by counsellors often have large files of notes denoting frequent attender behaviour at the GP's surgery, this has enormously important NHS resource implications, for example, as few as three per cent of patients who are frequent attenders consume 15 per cent of GP consultation time and even more resources of other kinds (Gill and Sharpe 1999).

A second side effect of a credible counselling service provision in primary care is the ubiquitous finding (not a conclusion but usually an incidental finding) from a large number of studies that the presence of such a service can considerably reduce community mental health team referrals as well as reduce referrals to psychiatric services by as much as 25 per cent. Furthermore, patients are seeking more appropriate, demedicalised, non-stigmatising forms of care which meet their needs and GPs are learning how to work collaboratively with practice counsellors (Somerset Health Authority 1996).

Finally, some counsellors working collaboratively with the GPs in primary health care teams have persuaded GPs to let them assess patients for whom the GP wishes to prescribe expensive anti-depressant medication. Instead, an in-depth assessment can inform the GP before expensive and possibly inappropriate decisions to prescribe are made. Counsellors with good assessment skills, used to working with depressed patients both on and off medication, can expect to save their entire salary out of reduced prescribing costs of anti-depressant medication (Heal 1997).

New drugs for the treatment of patients with depression are very expensive. This year, Serotonin Selective Re-Uptake Inhibitors (SSRIs) will cost the NHS slightly under £400m – approximately half of the entire deficit of health authorities and NHS trusts in the UK. To complicate matters a recent paper from the US suggests that only 20 per cent of their effect is an active drug effect, the rest being placebo and other effects, a very expensive placebo indeed (Kirsch and Sapirstein 1998).

To sum up, we have a competent workforce of practice counsellors struggling with sick, distressed and disturbed patients, some of them very sick, some very distressed and some very disturbed. The service they provide has a major impact on existing mental health and primary health care services.

Data now available from the preliminary analysis of the first datasets from the CORE Management System audit, evaluation and outcome project already shows that for many patients distress is often severe. The substantial overlap in levels of distress between primary care and tertiary level services indicates that only the 'worried well' are being seen by counsellors working in primary health care is a myth. From provisional data available it seems that at least 75 per cent of the patients seen are helped or greatly helped by seeing a counsellor (Mellor-Clarke *et al.* 2001).

What of the 25 per cent who are not? It is apparent that counsellors working in primary care have already unwittingly discovered that the supportive holding therapy they practice by seeing patients at longer intervals, making contact by telephone or letter, is remarkably effective at preventing further deterioration while these patients wait and wait and wait (if they are lucky) for their appointment with a more appropriate secondary tier service provider. Very few actually get worse.

In the absence in many parts of the UK of a credible secondary tier NHS service to whom these patients are referred and where they can be seen quickly, there is a myth that the counsellors return these patients to the GP for care on the grounds that he or she is much more experienced and skilled at looking after these patients than the counsellor. I use the word myth purposely because many counsellors know how daft is such a proposition.

Counsellors in primary care

Many counselling course trainees, some even in their first year of a diploma course, have found GP trainee placements in often precarious environments where they are sometimes poorly unsupported, unmanaged and often insecure. They are often exploited, their need for supervision seen by practice managers as a superfluous activity of the navel gazing kind. The placement provides a real baptism of fire, which could have potentially dangerous consequences to patients and counsellors alike.

Barely understood problems of patient management including confidentiality and other ethical problems frequently break to the surface for these students on placement. Patient disclosure of sexual abuse, criminal activity such as paedophile behaviour, violence and rape are not infrequently a part of the day-to-day work of trainee counsellors who may be unprotected by a practice mentor, an understanding practice manager or an aware GP, let alone a diploma training course provider.

To add to the problems, primary care counsellors working in the National Health Service come low down in the pecking order. Counsellors can be given two weeks notice of dismissal, suffer arbitrary pay cuts, ordered to stick to a six session limit, asked to provide full patient details to some distant NHS manager so that they can get paid and treated in ways that, by and large, not even contract cleaner services would put up with; that's only a few items from the exploitation list.

Furthermore, in almost every GP practice there is a 'Doubting Thomas' who thinks that counselling is a waste of time and loudly claims it is so. These critics usually arrive at coffee breaks or practice meetings triumphantly clutching the latest Bernard Manning type news story that rubbishes counselling.

Supervision and research into supervision in primary care

Having given a resumé of what is actually going on in the NHS and in primary care counselling, those who do not supervise counsellors working in primary care must be breathing a huge sigh of relief – thinking; 'How can they do it and how on earth could I provide expert supervision in such a demanding, high intensity environment?' There are those who do now realise why they feel so exhausted after a gruelling one and a half hour supervision session, where barely a quarter of the counsellor's current patient-load has been discussed and many of the problems presented seem insoluble.

However, research findings are now emerging from primary care about supervision both from what counsellors themselves have said and from what others who have studied supervision in this setting are reporting. In 1993 as part of the Counselling in Primary Care Trust's work identifying the training needs of counsellors working in primary care a counsellor survey was carried out using a one in ten sample from our counsellor database at the time (Einzig, Curtis Jenkins and Basharan 1995). All but one of the 24 counsellors in this small survey received supervision but only 4 of the 24 received payment for it from the practices in which they worked or received time off in lieu. All commented that in an ideal world they would have liked to have started work in a managed and supervised trainee placement and 2 of the 24 felt that their supervisor didn't seem to understand their needs in their work context. One added that this wasn't due to lack of skill or experience but lack of practical experience of the workplace of the GP counsellor.

As a result of this research a curriculum development project was commissioned which culminated in six University and College Masters Level One-Year Diploma programmes (and subsequently two-year degree programmes) supported by bursaries over three years. These courses offered the full range of modules identified by both the counsellors as necessary parts of their learning objectives and from the nation-wide consultation conducted by Penny Henderson who collated the findings and wrote the syllabus and curriculum specification for the course (Henderson 1994).

In the efforts to develop these educational programmes one vital part of the counsellors' practice, namely supervision, had been overlooked. Over time, counsellors and their supervisors shared their experiences in working together and it became apparent that a closer look at supervision was needed. It had already been identified that a shortage of skilled trained supervisors existed and that other NHS professionals had difficulty in understanding what supervision was and why counsellors needed it. In the light of these provisional findings an in-depth study of supervision in primary care was commissioned by the Counselling in Primary Care Trust (Burton, Henderson and Curtis Jenkins 1998).

Counselling supervision requirement is a uniquely British phenomenon and written into the codes of ethical practice of BAC and other counselling and psychotherapy organisations. As a result of the literature search it became apparent that there was much anecdotal, but limited empirical evidence of the impact of supervision on clinical practice. Some counsellors said that they learned more from personal therapy and supervision than from other parts of their training. However, in all the literature reviewed it was difficult to find studies that looked at the impact of supervision on clinical work and there were few studies of the experience of supervisees and their attitudes to supervision.

After an extensive literature review commissioned by The Counselling in Primary Care Trust and performed by Dr Mary Burton, 1500 books, book chapters, journal papers and articles were identified (available as a 22 page bibliography from the Counselling in Primary Care Trust). It was noted, like Carroll (1996), that the US literature concentrated on the multiplicity of theoretical models and the UK studies focused mainly on the actual day-to-day practice of supervision. Despite the enormous amount of writing available there appeared to be little empirical data available that could inform, for instance, purchasers and providers of the purpose of counselling supervision. Nor could it be used to inform them why they should not only insist that all counsellors have it but that it was part of the service that should be funded, not as an esoteric extra.

Supervision research project

It was then decided to concentrate the inquiry on the experiences of counsellors receiving supervision and a number of research questions were posed.

1. What is the impact of supervision on the clinical work of counsellors in primary care?

2. How well does supervision meet counsellors' needs at the moment?
3. What are counsellors' experienced difficulties with supervision?
4. How good is the 'match' between supervisors' and counsellors' theoretical orientations in primary care settings?
5. How satisfied are counsellors with their supervision?
6. How adequate is supervision in addressing problems unique to the primary care setting?

Efforts were concentrated on inquiring about:

- counsellor/supervisor congruence regarding theoretical stance and personal style
- positive and negative effects of supervision
- details of the problems of the setting identified by Hoag (1992) and others
- information about the supervision contract and about counsellor satisfaction
- counsellors' openness to learn
- impact of personal therapy on counselling practice
- the interface between personal therapy and practice supervision
- abusive supervisory relationships
- the 'impasse' described by Ruskin (1994).

In addition, a number of supervisors who were supervising GP counsellors were consulted.

A postal questionnaire was then constructed (questions were either left open or answered on a five point scale) and sent to two groups of GP counsellors. These two groups consisted of Group A, 65 recent graduates from the masters level diploma programmes in London, Bristol, Manchester and Strathclyde (with a 77 per cent response rate) and Group B, a one in ten random sample of 103 non diplomates taken from the name and address database maintained by the Counselling in Primary Care Trust. There was a 58 per cent response rate and respondents were matched by age, gender and locality.

Seven of the non-responders were either no longer working as counsellors (four), were currently not working because of health problems (one) or were otherwise unavailable (two). One respondent returned the questionnaire with a curt note wondering why the research had been commissioned, how the results would be published and asked to know the hidden agenda.

There were hardly any differences between the two groups. Sixty-three per cent worked only in primary care and several worked in more than one general practice.

What was learned from the results? First of all, it was apparent that there was a shortage of suitable supervisors. The supervisors in the study came from many professional backgrounds – social work, nursing, psychology and psychiatry as well as counselling. There were more female supervisors (72%) than male supervisors (8%). The male supervisors were mostly BAC (15%) or non-BAC accredited counsellors (22%) and psychotherapists (22%).

Twenty-two per cent of the supervisors had a masters degree, one in ten had a doctoral qualification and just under half had other unspecified qualifications. Only a quarter of the supervisors worked in primary health care as counsellors.

How 'matched' did the counsellors feel? The supervisors' theoretical orientations were predominantly psychodynamic or humanistic, and the counsellors' orientations were psychodynamic, humanistic or eclectic, which included Gestalt, TA, CAT, Jungian, Rogerian, person centred, psychosynthetic and integrative – a heady mix.

Yet, there was a highly significant correlation between counsellors and supervisors theoretical orientation ($p<0.003$). Counsellors tended to receive supervision from supervisors sharing the same core model. 'Mismatches' were seen sometimes as complementary but also as problematic. Attitudes to brief therapy (less of more) cognitive behaviour techniques (therapy by numbers), directiveness (un-person centred), willingness to see very disturbed patients and a closed interpersonal style were mentioned as causing difficulties.

How interested were the GPs in the practices in the supervision received by 'their' counsellors? Counsellors told us that the GPs 'rarely asked about it' and a few commented that 'they preferred it that way'. Just under half the counsellors were forced to pay for their supervision themselves, the rest was funded by their employers or the practices where they worked.

What did supervisors do, that is, how did they engage in supervision? Most used a discussion-based approach. Problem formulations, treatment plans or interpersonal process recall were rarely used nor were audio or video tapes. One supervisor directly observed the counsellor working, sitting in as a co-therapist on sessions.

A surprise finding was that over three-quarters of the counsellors recorded that their supervisor was trained in counselling supervision (the questionnaire failed to ask what the training consisted of) and just under three-quarters said that their supervisor 'was experienced in supervising counsellors who worked in primary care'. Eight out of ten supervisors were themselves receiving supervision for their supervisory practice. This compares with the more recent UK Survey of GP

Counsellors which found that 62 per cent reported that their supervisors were qualified in supervision and 20 per cent were not (Mellor-Clark *et al.* 2001).

Was supervision useful? Most of the counsellors rated the supervision they received as either very or extremely important but didn't answer the question of 'usefulness' directly. Common themes included support, containment, feedback, working with stuckness or difficulty, transference and countertransference issues, projective identification, premature interpretation and learning from mistakes. As one counsellor put it 'I get a fresh and objective view of each patient' and another 'to my surprise my supervisor focuses on the client'.

How well informed were counsellors about resources available for onward referral – a vital need given the complexity and severity of some patients' problems? A third reported lack of resources and lack of knowledge about the technical abilities of therapists in the private and NHS sectors.

Finally, what issues constantly cropped up in the counsellors' life that were presented in supervision? Only a third had dedicated office space, all had waiting lists which from the information derived from the National Counsellor Survey varied from 2 to 60 weeks from referral to assessment (mean = five weeks) and from assessment to counselling 0 to 100 weeks with a mean of 2.6 weeks (both vastly under the average waiting times in secondary and tertiary services).

Twenty-eight per cent used some form of patient audit (although the National Survey concluded that 18 per cent of counsellors collect no audit information at all). These audits mainly inquired about patient satisfaction (50%), goal attainment (30%) and only 14 per cent used previously published measures that would have allowed comparison of like with like.

Fifty per cent of respondents claimed to have adequate secretarial support. Less than half were allocated time to write up their records during their contracted hours and three-quarters recounted a major problem with patients they wished to refer on to more appropriate or more skilled service providers.

Overall, the counsellors in the research study expressed satisfaction with the supervision they received. They claimed to feel 'supported' and 'safe' in supervision. They commented about the interpersonal reflection of their work being the focus of their work in supervision.

There were, however, areas of dissatisfaction. Some counsellors noted that no written records were kept, that sometimes supervisors from a different theoretical persuasion actively criticised or failed to acknowledge the difference in approach, or that different therapeutic approaches had equal validity. Some were reported as failing to use parallel process effectively and did not try to bring to consciousness issues of countertransference.

Some claimed that supervisors did not 'speak up' for counsellors in service settings where the supervisor worked in a different (and often superior) position from the counsellor – and some counsellors commented on the tendency for a few supervisors to find difficulty in acknowledging their own areas of weakness or rigidity, a welcome sign that supervisors are mere humans, fallible and imperfect, even if the supervisee might want it otherwise.

Finally, one in ten described past abusive supervisory relationships – describing the use of supervisory material for the supervisor's gratification, rigid or authoritarian stance, pathologising the supervisee, giving consistent negative feedback, sexualisation of relationship, breaching boundaries and persistent lack of clarity about contracts.

Questions about personal therapy were also asked. Ninety-eight per cent of the correspondents had had personal therapy, 43 per cent in the past only and 47 per cent both in the past and currently. Most therapies were psychodynamic or humanistic with very few described as CBT, systemic, eclectic or brief. Successful personal therapy and the way it helped day-to-day working were very clear. Growth, self understanding and awareness, experience of being a client, working with one's own family issues, the recognition of transference and counter-transference, awareness of the process and very importantly an understanding of the power of the therapist and the capacity for good and evil were all recounted as positive effects. Finally, the experience of good therapy gave living proof that therapy does work.

A fifth of the counsellors identified negative effects of their own therapy on work with clients, a reminder that it's difficult working with one's own regression when a client is experiencing something similar and as one counsellor stated 'it brought up more than I could cope with which has sometimes left me in a place where it was very hard to be for my clients'.

The questionnaire also tried to tease out the boundary issues between counsellors and supervisors and results indicated that, for the most part, supervisors were scrupulous at maintaining the boundaries.

From the above what are the issues that should concern supervisors of counsellors in primary care? One conclusion is that supervisor accreditation seems to be an urgent requirement: within the NHS clinical governance framework this becomes essential. Counsellors may well overestimate the training their supervisors have received. 'Training', it appears, covers a wide area, a multiplicity of programmes and courses and workshops of varying quality, focus and length that urgently needs regulating.

Satisfaction levels were of course high. Perhaps this was an effect of the way some respondents saw the questionnaire itself as attacking them and their supervisors.

There clearly was dissatisfaction about supervisory practice which was lacking in teaching, suggesting reading, clarifying treatment goals and objectives (partly the effect of the medical workplace ethos), lack of attention to the counsellors' process in development, in dealing with impasses and the apparent frequency of abusive relationships particularly when a supervisor was provided as part of counselling service contract provision with the counsellor having no part in that decision. Non-disclosure by therapists in this situation was common as it was with trainees who feel out of their depth concealing their difficulties from supervisors. This could be due to shame and must be addressed.

A supervisory model working on the ideas of the late Viv Ball, Pat Fitzgerald (who at one time was the co-ordinator of the highly successful Derbyshire Primary Care Counselling Service) and Penny Henderson the Training Associate of The Counselling in Primary Care Trust and others has been outlined (Curtis Jenkins *et al.* 1997).

Elements within supervision of counsellors in primary care

It seem that one supervisor cannot fulfil all the roles and responsibilities asked of him or her. There are four distinct tasks in supervision. First of all there is the mentoring role, perhaps best fulfilled by the experienced counsellor already practising when the trainee or newly qualified counsellor starts work. This has worked well in the North and South Derbyshire services using a 'buddy' model with an experienced counsellor 'piggy backing' in the new counsellor and smoothing the way for a relatively stress free placement. This model was first described in the Nuffield Trust Project for Trainee General Practitioners in the 1960s which created the cadre of skilled and highly trained GP trainers and the current vocational training programmes for GPs in the UK. The modern GP registrar (as trainees are now called) is 'trained' in a way that most find supportive and enabling. It has also ensured that GP registrars in the UK are now probably the best prepared in the world for GP accreditation at the end of their two-year training programme.

A second task, good managerial supervision, is also essential. In some large well run often ex-fund holding practices, practice managers fill this role brilliantly. However, the management skills needed can vary widely. The task, the contract, the working conditions and the essential liaising with the rest of the primary health care team can be facilitated by a good sympathetic practice manager. The unsympathetic manager, with other agendas, can be almost completely disabling. Some counsellors, caught in such situations, have had to walk away rather than fight on in such unhappy workplaces.

The third task of supervision is casework consultation. The reality is all too often what family medicine in the US has called most graphically 'the corridor dump', the snatched consultation on the run between meetings, where GPs and counsellors frantically try to communicate and share in the frighteningly busy and often highly distressed environment of General Practice. It need not be like this. Encouraging consultant NHS psychotherapists to make themselves available for telephone consultation with counsellors has been very helpful. Where counsellors are managed by Mental Health NHS Trusts, regular and routine casework consultation often occurs. Some highly motivated psychiatrists have also made themselves available in this way. More formal meetings occur in some general practice settings where CPNs, psychologists and counsellors join in casework consultation about difficult or complex patients.

The fourth and final task is psychological supervision, which provides the full range of help to supervisees regarding clients, relationship with clients, interventions and so on.

It seems improbable that supervisors can necessarily fulfil all the other tasks at the same time. Without accurate and inside information it's often difficult for a supervisor to sense what actually goes on when a counsellor brings structural problems of service provision to supervision. Should these tasks be part of supervision anyway?

What are the solutions to the problems raised? First, counsellors starting work in primary healthcare need much more help in their undergraduate diploma training to prepare themselves to work in this testing environment. Training providers will soon discover that unmanaged trainee placements are no longer acceptable under the BAC code of practice and the proposed code of practice of CPC (the new association of counsellors and psychotherapists in primary care). Post-graduate masters level training provision that is tailored to the developmental and professional needs of counsellors working in primary health care is also urgently required. At present the position is unsatisfactory and still not meeting the needs of counsellors.

However, a number of initiatives across the UK are attempting to address this need.

There needs to be a commitment to build into counselling training a philosophy that the supervisor is perhaps the unseen other in every session. This ongoing dialogue is crucial to the maintenance and development of professional skill and expertise. It is unclear how often this is a reality. Many pick up what supervision is from experiencing it. It is also clear that urgent research is required to find out whether supervision really makes a difference – it is no longer acceptable to believe that this is a self-evident truth. The demand for evidence-based practice in modern healthcare ensures that someone, somewhere, sometime is bound to ask for such evidence. At the moment there are no convincing answers – at least not for NHS managers for whom the 'evidence' is the criteria on which all purchasing and provision of services is made.

Last, a story, a salutary reminder of the fragility of the foundations on which current supervision practice seems to be based. The Trust has supported a number of appropriate post-graduate trainings of counsellors in primary care. The diploma courses we supported with bursaries were originally planned to run for one year but were extended to two years and then to two plus one year masters degrees as time went by. The reasons were clear. It was considered unethical by the courses' consortium members to continue with the one-year format. Experience of student selection for these courses demonstrated that although most of the applicants arrived holding paper evidence of training and often glowing letters of support from supervisors, when these post graduate students joined the courses a few were relatively incompetent. The training and supervision references sometimes did not correlate at all with competence or incompetence. This caused great difficulties initially as the skill mix of the counsellors varied so widely that teaching became very difficult.

Subsequently some of the courses demanded audio or video evidence of clinical practice to help assess candidate suitability, rather than simply reports from supervisors (although the supervisors reports were still found to have value other than describing competence).

Conclusion

Briefly, and in conclusion, the following are thoughts and ideas to be borne in mind by supervisors of counsellors in primary care in the future.

1. Please start to think how you can incorporate these new or at least relatively new ideas in your workbox of supervision skills offered to counsellors.
2. Supervisors in the US are being sued on grounds of vicarious liability by the supervisees' clients. As a result, supervisors are having to change their supervisory practice, minimising risk by ensuring that the supervision does what it is meant to do to protect the client. What happens in the US today tends to happen in the UK tomorrow. There is a current potential liability of 2.5 billion dollars in legal claims against psychotherapists going through the courts in the US. The current potential claim liability for all the NHS is 2.5 billion pounds. It will happen here and it is only a question of time.
3. Supervisor training and accreditation need to be standardised and a level of 'good enough competence' established. Validation and certification procedures for working in specialist areas are urgently required.
4. Research needs to be carried out to find out what good supervision does. In the current climate it will come as no surprise if sceptical outsiders who hold the purse strings will say 'no proof – no money'.
5. Counselling training today needs to prepare counsellors to work in other environments besides private practice and to help them understand how they can gain acceptance if not mastery in their chosen

clinical settings. Supervisors have a responsibility to feed this back to counselling training providers.

6. How to use supervision effectively relies in part on supervisors teaching supervisees how the process works and what the rules are. Counsellors need to know what they can expect from supervision and to recognise bad supervision when they get it.
7. We need safeguards and quality assurance procedures with teeth. How easy is it for a supervisor to ensure that a supervisee stops work when distressed or temporarily unable to practice safely and effectively? How easy is it for a supervisor to ensure that incompetence is dealt with – not by supervisors struggling to improve counsellor competency levels through supervision when the counsellor concerned persistently presents the false self or remains convinced of their high clinical expertise in the face of evidence to the contrary?
8. We need to explain clearly and convincingly to NHS managers, GPs and others what supervision is and why it is so important.

I will end on a personal note. I have only mentored a small number of individual GP registrars when I worked as a GP trainer. Then I had no psychological supervision myself for the work I did. I still remember, with profound regret, how one of my GP registrars was damaged by my own mental state at the time when I was his mentor. At that time I was typically the last to realise how sick I was due to depression and how unfit I was to continue in my 'training' mentoring role let alone continuing to work as a GP. When I did and stopped work, I realised the damage was already done and my 'trainee' suffered. This can happen to supervisors too and appropriate mechanisms must be put in place to prevent such occurrences.

On a more positive note it is impressive to hear about the high quality of supervision many GP counsellors receive. Glowing reports about supervisors' unstinting support, concern for the individual and creativity, tact and ingenuity from counsellors working in the testing environment of primary care attest to this.

References

Baker, R., Allen, H., Gibson, S., Newth, J. and Baker, E. (1998) 'Evaluation of a primary care counselling service in Dorset.' *British Journal of General Practice 48*, 1049–1053.

Burton, M., Henderson, P. and Curtis Jenkins, G. (1998) 'Primary care counsellors' experience of supervision.' *Counselling 9*, 2, 122–133.

Carroll, M. (1996) *Counselling Supervision: Theory, Skills and Practice.* London: Cassell.

Curtis Jenkins, G. (1999) 'Collaborative care in the United Kingdom.' *Clinics in Office Practice 26*, 2, 411–412. London: WB Saunders Company.

Curtis Jenkins, G., Burton, M., Henderson. P., Foster. J. and Inskipp, F. (1997) *Supervision of Counsellors in Primary Care. Supplement No. 3.* Staines: Counselling in Primary Care Trust Publications.

Einzig, H., Curtis Jenkins, G. and Basharan, H. (1995) 'The training needs of counsellors in primary medical care.' *Journal of Mental Health 4*, 204–209.

Gill, D. and Sharpe, M. (1999) 'Frequent consulters in general practice. A systematic review of studies of prevalence associations and outcome.' *Journal of Psychosomatic Research 47*, 2, 115–130.

Heal, M. (1997) 'Introducing a counselling culture to general practice.' *Journal of the Institute of Counselling and Psychotherapy 6*, 15–19.

Henderson, P. (1994) *Counselling in Primary Healthcare Diploma.* Staines: Counselling in Primary Care Trust.

Hoag, L. (1992) 'Psychotherapy in the general practice surgery. Considerations of the frame.' *British Journal of Psychotherapy 8*, 4, 417–429.

Howard, K. I., Orlinsky, D. E. and Jueger, R. J. (1999) 'Clinically relevant outcome research in individual psychotherapy. New models to guide the researchers and the clinician.' *British Journal of Psychiatry 165*, 4–8.

Kirsch, I. and Sapirstein, G. (1998) 'Listening to prozac but hearing placebo. A meta analysis of anti depressant medication.' *Prevent and Treatment 1*, article 002a. APA Publication.

Mellor-Clark J., Simms Ellis, R. and Burton, M. (2001) *National Survey of Counsellors Working in Primary Care. Evidence for Growing Professionalisation.* (Submitted for publication.)

Ruskin, R. (1994) 'When Supervision may fail.' In S. E. Greben and R. Ruskin (eds) *Clinical Perspectives on Psychotherapy Supervision.* Washington: American Psychiatric Press.

Somerset Health Authority (1996) *The Cost Effectiveness of Introducing a Counselling Service into the Primary Care Setting in Somerset.* Taunton: Somerset Health Authority.

Chapter 9

Supervision in Primary Care

Corset or Camisole?

Rita Arundale

Introduction

Over the past several years counselling in primary care has increased dramatically. In Teesside alone, 85 per cent of GP practices have one or more counsellors as part of the team, with clients generally having access to more than one counselling orientation. Because of this increase the need for appropriate supervision for counsellors in primary care has risen accordingly. It has been necessary, therefore, for supervisors to expand their knowledge of the primary care system, its foibles, peculiarities, strengths and weaknesses (Corney and Jenkins 1993), in order to offer supervisees an informed and professional service which reflects familiarity with the environment in which they practice. Supervisors expect supervisees to have intimate knowledge of the workings of the primary care system as well as the ability to integrate this knowledge into an already established, and occasionally, hostile group setting. Encouraging supervisees to work through the dynamics of these relationships and establishing a professional counselling service is a valuable part of the supervisory process.

Supervisors are used to viewing the primary care environment once removed, that is through the eyes and reports of the counsellor (East 1995). It is easy for them, from this vantage point, to deflect attention away from their own thoughts, prejudices and beliefs about primary care. Safely cocooned in this supervisory role it is all too easy to concentrate on their supervisees' inner world without including the external world of primary care. On the other hand, supervisors are challenged to open themselves to the ever-changing face of the counselling profession and the increasing demands made upon primary care counsellors for evaluation, audit and the development of a professional identity.

What, for example, are supervisors' views about expanding the role of counselling in primary care? Are supervisors stuck in the old routine of seeing the counsellor as someone who goes to the surgery, sees referred clients and then disappears into the ether until the next session day at the GP practice? Many surgeries still work on this principle not only with counsellors but also with other disciplines, making it difficult to envisage a time when counsellors might be accepted as an integral part of the primary care team. Other GP practices are willing to adopt a more flexible policy towards the counselling service and openly seem to value the work of the counsellor through invitations to team meetings and social occasions as well as providing the opportunity to educate team colleagues about counselling. Furthermore, this offers an opening for counsellors to be educated in turn by exposure to how other disciplines work and integrate counselling into a multi-disciplinary mileau.

Interesting questions being posed by counsellors and supervisors in the present uncertain climate include:

- are supervisors aware of the implications for the counsellor of the Government's policy on primary care groups (PCGs)?
- what will happen if the new PCGs decide to opt for a less-than-adequate counselling service in general practice (that is, less than that defined by the counselling in medical settings division of the BAC 1998)?
- how do counsellors/supervisors define their professional identity within the PCG system?
- will counsellors/supervisors integrate themselves within mental health teams or will they stand alone?
- how is the learning of supervisees best facilitated around these issues?

The medical profession, by tradition, mainly uses a biomedical approach, each illness or disease being treated in isolation and the needs of the person being second to that of the illness being treated. Using a biopsychosocial model (Engel 1980), wherein the whole person, including their social and environmental concerns is considered when treatment is being planned, is slowly becoming more acceptable within the medical profession. Because of this, counsellors are in a unique position to promote the holistic treatment of patients by integration within the primary care team. They can offer complementary treatment strategies, open up the possibility of a more equitable service (Whitehead 1994) and broaden their role through early psychological intervention for physical illness, life changes as well as the more standard psychological presenting issues. Being aware of changing trends and encouraging and supporting supervisees in developing a professional approach becomes a key challenge for supervisors. This would incorporate not only the techniques and tools of counselling but also the political awareness which will allow counsellors to take their place within the mental health profession, secure in their understanding of the issues under discussion becomes a key challenge for supervisors.

Supervisors need to scrutinise their own philosophy and beliefs about their role as supervisors to see where they stand in the light of a patient's right to be consulted at every stage of their treatment and in encouraging and supporting supervisees in their role as primary care counsellors.

Often counsellors are flying in the face of tradition, perhaps asking the doctor to suspend medication or find an alternative treatment, on the basis of their assessment. This is no light achievement, requiring courage and determination, a belief in themselves and the counselling process. Supervisors seek to encourage supervisees to find their own level of skill, influence and power within the practice team. Supporting and affirming counsellors while enabling their awareness of learning and developmental needs (Carroll 1996) is an acquired skill on the part of supervisors and nowhere is it more needed than when supervising counsellors in primary care. When working within primary care the specific ramifications of that environment are more than usually apparent (Corney and Jenkins 1993). These ramifications include supporting counsellors in setting up a secure environment for their clients if the environment is constantly in a state of change and encouraging counsellors to respond when faced with the fact that the counselling room can change from week to week or be commandeered without prior notice.

Primary care counsellors do not have the luxury of the tailored environment of private practice. More time needs to be spent on processing the environment with primary care supervisees than with those in private practice.

Working in primary care is not just about appearing at the GP practice, seeing clients and leaving the surgery. It is also about incorporating the service into the practice, using education to demonstrate what counselling can achieve in co-operation with the other team members. It means offering and promoting the strengths of counselling as opposed to the traditional methods of treatment and showing how counselling can enhance the service offered by the primary care team.

The current trend in health care is on auditing and evaluating the service provided. Funding bodies are unwilling to spend money on services which cannot in some way prove themselves to be effective. Because of this supervisors need to ask about the implications of auditing and evaluation for themselves, about current research studies and methodologies, about evaluating and auditing their own work as supervisors, about to whom they are accountable, about their competency to supervise counsellors in auditing and evaluating and indeed, about whether or not supervisors should supervise in this particular area.

These are only a few of the many focus-points relevant to the present situation. Qualitative evaluation of a counselling service has always been seen as the most difficult area to audit, and yet for our own sakes and the sake of the counselling profession, we need to grasp and shape the evaluation methods to our needs. It is easy to get caught up in the restrictive methods proposed by well meaning but essentially administrative bodies who do not fully understand the nature of the counselling profession and its process.

The Primary Care Setting

Effective supervisors consider their relationship to primary care, not at one-remove from the system, but face to face, and ask a number of questions in relation to their understanding of the supervisory role within the primary care system. One way is to think of a line with supervisor, counsellor and primary care written on it, as below:
and consider whether supervisors use counsellors as buffers between themselves and primary care. Removing the word 'counsellor' from the line, as shown below,

SUPERVISOR ------------ COUNSELLOR ------------ PRIMARY CARE

leaving only 'supervisor' and 'primary care' causes supervisors to be faced with a new reality.

SUPERVISOR ----------------------- PRIMARY CARE

Supervisor reactions to this new reality can include feeling vulnerable, confused, chaotic, fearful and exposed. Many don't understand the context of primary care and focus on issues such as the need for a three-cornered contract or, I hope, feel responsible and spend more time on investigating the impact of primary care on clinical work.

When considering how they think about themselves in relation to primary care, supervisors will take into account:

- the size of the practice (6000+ patients is the usual number of patients per surgery)
- the role of team working
- what is funded and by whom
- management of the practice
- any needs for audit of clinical work.

Many supervisors do not understand the old primary care system, with fundholding and non-fundholding practices, and are confused about the new primary care commissioning system. A book explaining the new system would be helpful as would be a consistent primary care system across the whole country. The system of auditing can also be rigid and counsellors may be expected to compromise confidentiality by having to give names of clients, or more. There may be a need for more interfacing between funding agencies and counselling services to highlight this anomaly.

Corset or camisole?

This chapter was entitled 'Corset or camisole' in order to highlight the restrictions and boundaries imposed in the primary care environment. Compared and contrasted they raise many issues for supervisors:

Corset

1. Work that is time-limited – six to eight sessions irrespective of client needs.
2. No audit – no funds.
3. Management of client caseload which challenges the counsellor's autonomy as a practitioner.
4. Pressure from waiting lists.
5. Pressure of the medical model and how treatment is viewed by both health professionals and patients and what the patients' expectations are when they come to the practice for help.
6. Over-zealous use of confidentiality – the counsellor's self-imposed 'corset'.

Camisole

1. Provides access to counselling for many people who would miss out because of the short contracts (six to eight sessions).
2. It is more acceptable, appropriate and less stigmatising to see a counsellor than to be referred to secondary care.
3. When counselling provision works well it works very well.
4. The counsellor works in a professional manner, within practice guidelines which are often unwritten. If the structure is good and the organisation is well thought out, the counsellor is more likely to be respected as a professional and the flexibility will be more in evidence.
5. The opportunity of working within the practice guidelines and procedures and promotes healthy relationships between counsellors and other health professionals.

It is interesting that a corset can be supportive when someone has a bad back. A parallel can be drawn here in that if an organisation's structure or 'back bone' is weak and has little support, then there are usually many guidelines and rules to contain the organisation but little flexibility. However if an organisation is well structured, guidelines are what they suggest they are, guidelines, and a degree of flexibility is enabled.

Supervisors who work, or are thinking of working, in primary care are invited to consider the following.

1. That counselling in primary care is free, provides a broad access to clientele, it is available in a crisis or when the client/patient is desperate, it prevents referral to a psychiatrist and provides an opportunity for a psychological response to physical presentations.
2. That supervising counsellors in primary care has its peculiarities. The contract with the organisation is complex, the supervisor may have only a supporting role to justify their place in the organisation, and there may be no consistent agency structure.
3. That supervisors need to position themselves in relation to the primary care system and determine whether they are integrated into it or isolated. Most supervisors feel isolated, but may find a voice now in the new re-organisation.
4. That they have to determine what is their responsibility as a supervisor to the primary care agency. Most supervisors would answer that they are there to ensure the safety and the quality of counselling work for the patient and the practice.
5. That there may come a time when they would contact the practice. If the counsellor needs support for a complex problem, if there is the possibility of dangerous or unethical work by counsellors or when the supervisee is in a training organisation there are possible scenarios when the supervisor would contact the practice.
6. That the boundaries of communication between professionals needs to be considered. Are there any? Confidentiality needs to be negotiated with the client's consent, as the primary care setting is a multi-disciplinary one.
7. That the broader picture of primary care and the expanding role of counselling within the confines of the primary care parameters requires attention. Counsellors are being asked to justify their employment in this setting and they need to be familiar with qualitative and quantitative outcome measures for counselling in primary care, and may

want to challenge the assumptions of the randomised control trial. Counsellors and supervisors should be recording their interventions and treatment plans and be willing to publish in medical journals. Counselling trainers should be challenged about counselling placements in GP surgeries, where tighter guidelines and boundaries are necessary. Training for brief therapy is also useful.

8. That supervisors need to review how active they ought to be in the political scene. If not, why not, and how do they imagine developing political awareness would affect their roles and relationships with supervisees? If yes, how has this affected their role?

The political scene is a minefield of misinformation and speculation in the light of current government proposals. While it may be desirable, it is a considerable task to integrate all the information and make useful sense of it at present. But it remains important to be active, involved and aware of what is happening in the political arena.

Conclusion

The restrictions which abound within the health care system, and primary care in particular, are often viewed as extreme and are adhered to in a way which may not allow counsellors to exert as much autonomy as they might like. One reason for so many restrictive guidelines is the fear that many health professionals feel in relation to counselling. They do not understand the process and therefore feel the need to contain the 'beast' in order to control it.

Too much emphasis is often placed on working within the guidelines at the cost of clients' needs. After all, if a patient had a wound which needed dressing and was referred to the practice nurse, would the GP place a restriction on the number of times the wound had to be dressed? If the wound was not healed within those times, would the GP refuse further dressings, or would he/she trust the practice nurse to know when the wound was healed or needed further treatment? In the same way counsellors need to have the authority and flexibility, within the guidelines, to know when to step outside them for the well-being of the client. To be able to discuss these needs with the doctor/team, and to have the confidence to assert their professional opinion and preferred treatment strategy is extremely important.

It is the duty of supervisors to support supervisees in developing these skills. Supervision as a profession also needs to keep pace with the growth of the therapeutic profession in primary care, and in order to do this it is not only desirable but essential that supervisors increase their knowledge of the systemic and political background of the primary care environment.

References

BAC (1998) *Guidelines for the Employment of Counsellors in General Practice.* Rugby: BAC.

Carroll, M. (1996) *Counselling Supervision: Theory, Skills and Practice.* London: Cassell.

Corney, R. and Jenkins, R. (1993) (eds) *Counselling in General Practice.* London: Routledge.

East, P. (1995) *Counselling in Medical Settings.* Buckingham: Open University Press.

Engel, G. L. (1980) 'The clinical application of the biopsychosocial model.' *American Journal of Psychiatry 137,* 5, 535–544.

Whitehead, M. (1994) 'Equity issues in the NHS: who cares about equity in the NTIS?' *British Medical Journal 308,* 1284–1287.

Further reading

Atkinson, C. and Hayden, J. (1992) 'Managing change in primary care: strategies for success.' *British Medical Journal 304,* 1488–1490.

Balint, M. (1957) *The Doctor, his Patient and the Illness.* Kent: Pitman Medical Publishing.

Feltham, C. and Dryden, W. (1994) *Developing Counsellor Supervision.* London: Sage.

Illich, I. (1976) *Limits to Medicine. Medical Nemesis: The Expropriation of Health.* London: Marian Boyars.

McLeod, J. (1994) *Doing Counselling Research.* London: Sage.

Robson, C. (1993) *Real World Research.* Oxford: Blackwell.

Chapter 10

Supervision in Primary Care
What is in the Kitbag?

Jane Rosoman

Introduction

Over many years working as a counsellor in primary care I have collected many ideas, questions and exercises that have proved themselves useful to a practitioner in this field. Hence the metaphor of the 'kitbag' in the title. Coming as they do from all sorts of different orientations and ways of working, the contents of the kitbag have little coherence or co-ordination. In fact the kitbag has become very heavy and definitely in need of 'sorting out'. Preparation for this chapter took the form of 'clearing my counselling clutter', that is, trying to develop some coherence for my work as a supervisor working in primary care. Doing this forced me to isolate what are the essential tasks for the supervisor in this context.

These essentials focus on some questions facing supervisors of counsellors in primary care:

1. What is the influence of the context of primary care on the work of supervision?
2. What language is used within primary care, how does it shape what is done and what takes place in supervision?
3. What is being integrated in the supervision of counsellors working in primary care?

Context

Primary care is in turbulence. This is mainly due to two influences: the reorganisation of GP practices into primary care groups and the end of fundholding. The future of counselling in primary care looks uncertain as each primary care group makes its own decisions on how to allocate its budget (Curtis

Jenkins, Chapter 8). At the same time primary care counsellors are talking among themselves and beginning to establish a professional organisation to represent their interests. The uneasy tensions within each group are mirrored and reflected back in the concerns of GPs, counsellors and patients or clients. This is an example of the context influencing supervision: holding and examining this anxiety is a requirement of supervision. The dilemma for supervisors is how to enable counsellors to manage all these concerns and still have time and energy for the myriad issues that are brought by clients. Counsellors are asked to hold huge amounts of primitive anxiety which come from clients, from colleagues and from the community at large. All three of these groups project their concerns on to medical systems. This is an another example of the influence of the context on supervision. Because the process is largely unconscious, it does not get much acknowledgement.

Linking to this is narrative and its use in therapy. Work with clients in primary care often feels more like a conversation with some therapeutic intent or meaning rather than conventional counselling (McLeod 1997). Such conversations highlight the differences in the language we use when we belong to a health care system. When we belong to a counselling system these differences can make communication between the two systems difficult, for example, the impact of the word 'patient' in contrast to the word 'client' for supervisors and counsellors.

Language

Focusing on language and how it influences what is done has emerged from both family therapy and brief solution focused therapy. Since the setting in which they work is imbued with the medical model, assessment, diagnosis and treatment as well as notions of illness primary care, counsellors need to be alert to the language they use. Certain 'schools' within counselling and psychotherapy are more aligned with the medical model than others. Recent developments in systemic therapies, with their emphasis on language and interaction and the construction of social meanings, have challenged the helping professions. The writings of O'Hanlon and Beadle (1997) and White (1996) explore these themes with humour and integrity.

Primary care counselling offers clients opportunities to tell their stories. Narrative therapy and its emphasis on language and the way problems are framed gives counsellors the opportunity to bring new possibilities into the stories told by clients. These stories focus on the future rather than the past and help people reconnect with a sense of hope and possibility, bringing new insights which reframe old problems. As always, the process is about validating the clients' felt experience and their ideas about their lives, while at the same time ensuring possibilities for change are discovered and amplified.

Integration

In attempting to develop coherence about what it is essential to integrate in primary care supervision, a map was needed. Triangles provided such an image. Why this shape? A convinced systemic thinker might well have expected to use circles. However, two reasons influenced the decision to use triangles rather than circles. First, triangles and triangular relationships are so often a feature in family therapy. Second, the thinking of the Tavistock Institute of Marital Studies, and in particular, Janet Mattinson who has published her thoughts on triangles in *The Reflection Process in Casework Supervision* (1975) and *Mate and Stalemate* (1978), have been very influential in the field of supervision.

In supervision, it is difficult to pay attention to more than two points of focus and yet it is often the third point that holds the issues requiring attention and that are being ignored or denied. This third point may well contain anxiety and be troublesome to both counsellor and client, and indeed the supervisor. However, it is the supervisor's job to ensure all points of the triangle are considered. Not to do so may mean the spectre of unsafe practice looms larger. Keeping triangles in mind gives freedom to play within the supervisory relationship and to ensure that all three corners are looked at. Indeed it is an important feature of supervision to pay attention to each point, but not in a dogmatic way. Supervision has to be creative and not formulaic. The kitbag provided nine very familiar triangles.

While noticing the language they use, supervisors need to consider what is in their kit bags and what they are choosing to integrate with what. Implicit in supervision in primary care, is a focus on the speed of change and the demands of counsellors in primary care. Some supervisors are unaware of the extent of the changes and imminent deadlines facing counsellors in this context. Others may feel swamped with anxiety and it is important to allow space for exploring these concerns and for sharing information. In addition it is necessary to sort out the differences between counselling in primary care and supervision in this setting. To clarify this and to be able to differentiate between the two processes is valuable learning and enables them to move ahead with supervision.

The response to the ideas about triangles is usually enthusiastic and supervisors can come up with several more which can be important to their own practice.

Much discussion focuses on the difficulty of keeping the three points of the triangle in mind and how often the trap of only paying attention to two corners can catch supervisors. An example of this is the debate between longer-term work and brief work in the context of primary care. There are those who insist brief work is the only way to counsel in primary care and exclude any consideration of the value of long term work. More unusual is the primary care counsellor who only does long-term work and who does not consider the value of brief interventions. Holding in mind the three corners of the triangle, assessment, brief work and longer term work ensures the client's needs are considered as well as the demands of the setting, and reinforces the belief that assessment is the foundation of good practice.

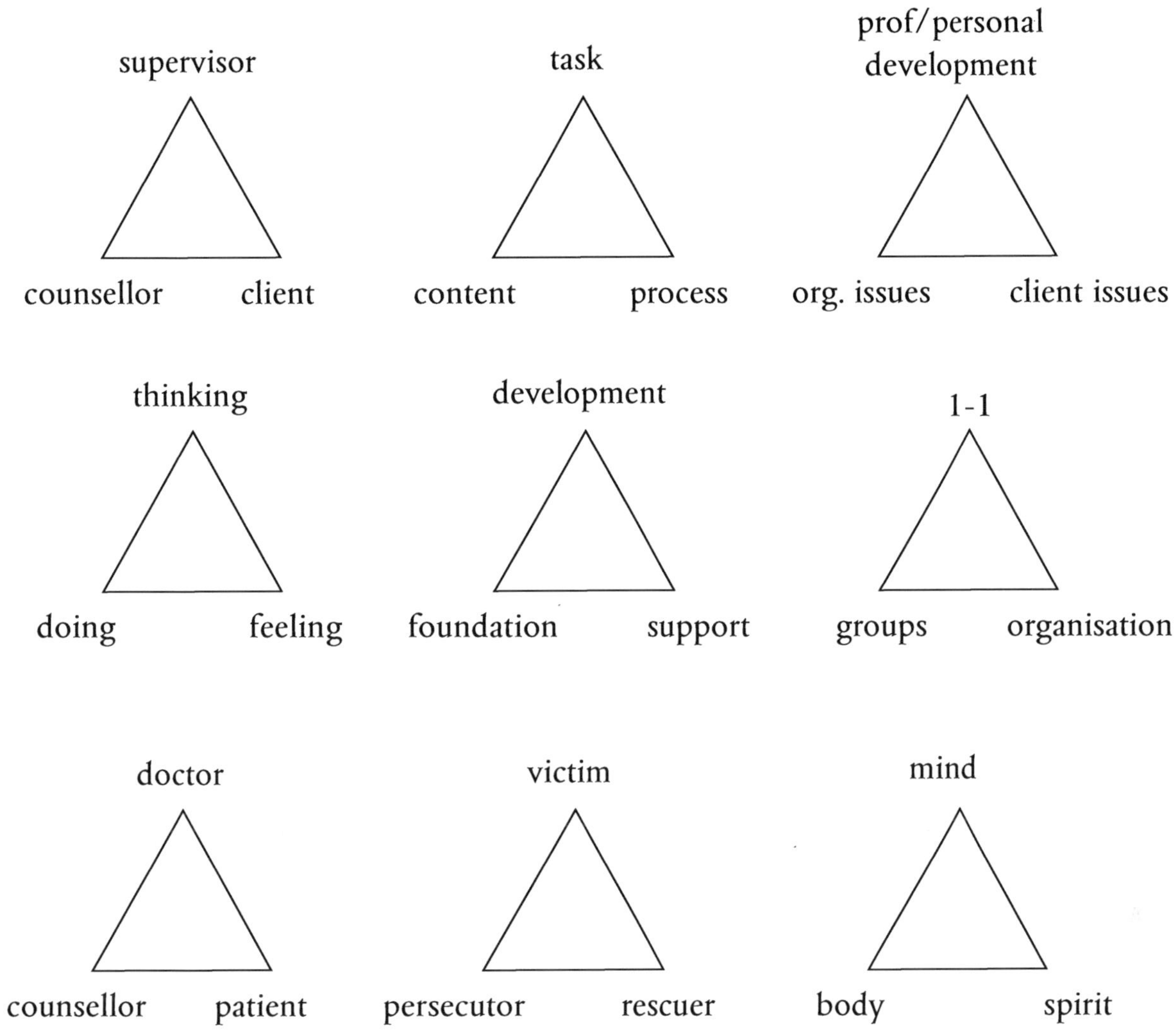

Figure 10.1: Triangles representing themes that may emerge through supervision

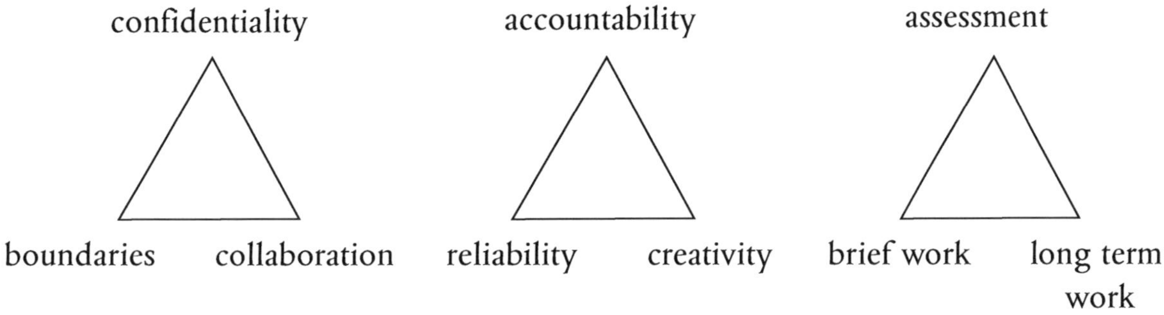

Figure 10.2: More examples of triangles representing supervisory issues

One triangle that generates a lot of energy and enthusiasm is the 'mind-body-spirit', with its concentration on how often the spirit is neglected in medical settings. Some medical practitioners distance themselves from complementary therapies while others have successfully integrated yoga and massage into their practices. In primary care, staff need help and support to do their work well.

Conclusion

This chapter highlights the importance of context and the impact it has on counselling and the supervisory process. Health care organisations have needs too. Uncertainty and turbulence remain a hook that catches a supervisor and can become a key feature threatening to fill the time allotted to supervision. Parallel process issues enter our work, particularly in terms of energy levels and in the dilemmas which are presented. Of some importance too is the fact that men can be left out when gender issues are not held in mind (could this be another triangle?). Apparently a geodesic sphere, that is a structure made out of triangles, is the strongest, most flexible structure known to engineers and architects. How apt a model for supervisors, who need all the strength and flexibility they can get!

References

McLeod, J. (1997) *Narrative and Psychotherapy.* London: Sage.

Mattinson, J. (1975) *The Reflection Process in Casework Supervision.* London: Tavistock Institute of Marital Studies.

Mattinson, J. (1978) *Mate and Stalemate.* London: Tavistock Institute of Marital Studies.

O'Hanlon, W. and Beadle, S. (1997) *A Field Guide to Possibility Land.* London: BT Press.

White, M. (1996) *Re-authoring Lives: Interviews and Essays.* Adelaide: Dulwich Centre Press.

Further reading

Hughes, L. and Pengelly, P. (1997) *Staff Supervision in a Turbulent Environment.* London: Jessica Kingsley Publishers.

Chapter 11

Food as Metaphor or as Nutrition

Supervising in Eating Disorders

Margaret Tholstrup

Introduction

Working with clients in any psychological setting will at some time present ethical issues for both counsellor and supervisor. When the client abuses food, ethical issues become even more complex: the potential now exists that the psychological work will transgress what is normally a clear boundary between the provision of emotional care and of physical or physiological care. If the client is in the habit of abusing food by abstaining, bingeing, vomiting, over-eating compulsively or any combination of these, she will resort to these behaviours and increase their frequency and intensity when the feelings that this behaviour has masked start to emerge in the counselling. This puts her physical health at risk; indeed anorexia and bulimia are among the very few fatal mental conditions, whether death is caused as a consequence of the behaviour with food (such as a heart attack due to long-term potassium deficiency) or as a consequence of the abuse (for example, depression leading to suicide). The client who reports that she is resorting to food to deal with emerging, difficult-to-cope-with feelings faces the counsellor with the following dilemma:

> Does the counsellor interpret the eating behaviour in psychological terms, using the stories and descriptions of the client's eating patterns as metaphors for what and how the client is feeling; or does she confront the eating behaviour directly, holding in mind that this behaviour is a form of self-harm and the client is putting her physical health at risk?

This overlap between physical and psychological care places both counsellor and supervisor in a unique position vis-à-vis the safe and ethical practice of both counselling or psychotherapy and of supervision.

The aim of this chapter is to highlight the impact of these issues on supervision and the supervisory relationship. It will also ask questions to help supervisors clarify their own feelings about food and their role when their supervisee's client uses food, not as a method of nutrition, but as a metaphor for unexpressed feelings. Some of the areas discussed will include:

- what is the role of the supervisor in this situation?
- what is his responsibility to the counsellor and to the client?
- where and with whom does the boundary of safe practice and responsibility lie?
- how does he (the supervisor) help the counsellor deal with the threat to the client's physical health?
- who holds responsibility for confronting these behaviours?
- what issues does this dilemma raise for the counsellor?
- how much of the acting-out through food is confronted in the consulting room?
- is it safe and ethical practice for the counsellor to address the client's behaviour around food?
- is it safe and ethical practice for the counsellor not to address the client's behaviour around food?

Eating disorders

For much of the time for most people, food is a method of nutrition, be it a sandwich gobbled during a quick lunch break or a biscuit with coffee to stave off hunger pangs before the next scheduled meal. Food is also the central focus or even the excuse for people to congregate formally or informally, from a business breakfast through lunch in the cafeteria with colleagues to groups of friends sharing a kitchen supper in the evening. Food provides the focal point of major celebrations, from a major life transition (baptism, bar mitzvah, wedding, funeral) to the holiday markers which divide up the calendar year (Passover, Thanksgiving, Ramadan, Christmas) where particular food, or its absence, takes on symbolic meaning. Our language is rife with similes and metaphors involving food and eating; for example, 'As American as apple pie' which evokes the image of Mom in a gingham apron, flour up to her elbows, surrounded by her loving family, putting a steaming apple pie on to the table in a warm kitchen full of luscious and enticing smells. For some reason this image represents archetypal Americana, though obviously it is not only Americans who bake and enjoy eating fresh hot apple pie.

Food is central to our most primal need for survival, as it is with all living creatures; without it we starve and die, thereby ceasing to exist. The provision of sustenance is also essential for human psychological development; the way in which a mother responds to her infant's cries for food and how she holds her infant while feeding it has a considerable impact of how he develops as a person. In *Body Self and Psychological Self*, Krueger (1989) writes about how the infant develops its ego and subsequently a sense of self:

> Bodily experiences and sensations, internal and surface, form the core around which the ego develops. As the kinesthetic body boundaries are being determined, an important parallel process occurs with psychic boundary formation and functioning ... The subjective reality testing of what is inside and outside the body has a psychological counterpart in the distinction between self and nonself. Accurate, consistent perceptions of body self, psychological self and their interaction are necessary to a cohesive sense of self. (p.4)

This interweaving of the physical and psychological becomes less pronounced as the child develops the capacity to translate internal sensations into verbal representations;

> ...[with the development of a sense of verbal self]...they [infants] now have the psychic mechanisms and operations to share their interpersonal world knowledge and experience, as well as to work on it in imagination or reality (Stern 1985, p.167).

Bruch (1979) was the first to hypothesise that the person with an eating disorder never completes this transition successfully, remaining trapped in a confusion between what is psychological and what is physical. Feelings are therefore expressed via food which is avoided or gorged upon, then held on to in order to fill an internal void or forcefully ejected via vomiting or purging. Food is desperately craved and desperately feared, yet the bottom line is that it is essential for life, so can never be totally given up as can be other substances frequently misused (alcohol, drugs, smoking) as a substitute for feelings. This presents the counsellor and therefore the supervisor with the difficult dilemma as to how much and whether to confront the eating behaviour being used as a metaphor for feelings.

My interest and enthusiasm for the subject comes from working in the field for ten years, five as a therapist in an out-patient eating disorders unit and more recently in independent practice. The chapter will include some exercises which will help the supervisor clarify his or her own issues and reactions to food and eating behaviour, with the hope that they will continue to debate and discuss the questions raised for supervision of counselling when the client the supervisee brings has an eating disorder.

Food as metaphor

As mentioned above, food and eating are very emotive subjects for everyone, including the supervisor, and are frequently used or abused in times of stress. This is a common experience for everyone, and it is important for the supervisor to identify their own behaviour with food when they are stressed. Most will agree that they do behave differently towards food when they are stressed. This helps to establish the strong link between food and feelings and helps the supervisor learn more about him or herself. This serves to break down a potential her-and-me split when the supervisee describes a client's eating behaviour.

The way to enter into the world of the eating disordered client more graphically is to explore how the client uses food as a metaphor. The experience, however, is physical or physiological and highlights the way in which the client uses food as a metaphor. Imagine eating a tub of yoghurt, an apple and a banana and thinking of it as the total intake for the day (this is the regular diet of one of my clients, excluding vomited binges and coffees). The supervisor is urged to consider their responses to the following questions:

- how would you feel if this is all you ate in a day?
- or if this is all you ate every day?
- if, after eating this, you took a handful of laxatives?

Reactions and responses will be very illuminating. The supervisor will probably feel hungry, ill and quite desperate, and be taken aback by the small quantity of food this represents. It will probably be very different from their normal diet. Allowing oneself the visual representation has quite a different impact from that of a hypothetical discussion about the quantity of food consumed and exaggerates even further how merged are the client's experiences of psychological and physical needs for food.

Repeating this with different types of food frequently binged on, such as a bag of mini Mars bars, individual packets of crisps or a loaf of bread (sliced and in a bag), elicits information of a different kind:

- how would the supervisor feel if they were to eat an entire bag of mini Mars bars, 12 small packets of crisps, followed by the loaf of bread as a snack?
- then went into the bathroom and threw it all up?
- then started all over again?

The graphic representation of the food followed by the description of the subsequent behaviour makes a considerable impact on everyone, and the supervisor may feel sickened and quite ill at the idea of consuming so much food all at once. For some eating the pile of chocolate or that many bags of crisps might be possible. However, the concept of actually eating this much regularly followed by throwing up just to repeat the experience is usually more than anyone wants to contemplate. From this exercise emerges an awareness of the desperation and shame that the person behaving in this way must feel as well as their conflicted attitude towards food. It also identifies the echo between feelings and what is being acted out with the food. That this is actually dangerous behaviour with physical sequelae is obvious: in all the above examples the client is not eating and holding on to sufficient food to nourish her body and provide the vital nutrients she needs to function in a healthy way. She is also jeopardising her health; this is a very important point to bear in mind.

The second point is the moot question as to whether the client is able to understand and use psychological interventions and support if her brain is deprived of essential nutrients, her body hurts and she is obsessed with the thought of food. If the client is abstaining or bingeing and vomiting, is she making appropriate use of the counselling time dedicated to her? Abusing food outside of sessions represents her difficulty in holding on to feelings and bringing them to the counselling sessions. This thought is often a new revelation to supervisors who may never have considered this possibility.

Food as nutrition

How willing are counsellors to weigh clients or advise them on their nutritional intake? Few counsellors would consider it an appropriate task or part of their contract with the client. This presents the counsellor with a dilemma: in order for the client to get better both physically and psychologically, someone needs to assume this responsibility. Food must be removed as a substitute for feelings and become solely a method of nutrition while the counsellor focuses on the meaning of food as a metaphor. Just as a functioning, healthy adult is able to differentiate between food and feelings, between physical and psychological needs, so the eating disordered client needs someone (or two people) to care for both aspects of her eating disorder: without someone to address food issues, the psychological work may fail. Working in a hospital environment as I did in an outpatient eating disorders service makes resolving this dichotomy easier, with one person (myself) taking responsibility for both aspects. In my independent practice with this client group and depending on the severity of the problem, I will share the responsibility with a nutritionist.

Case example

A counsellor brings the following excerpt from a client statement to supervision:

> I am so big – just look at my thighs and my hips – I am huge! These jeans are so tight at the waist compared to yesterday – I am sure I've put on at least five pounds. That's probably because last night I ate five bagels as well as my usual

> vegetables, threw everything up then went out and bought more food just to binge on and threw that up. It's all that food I ate that has put on all this weight.

What is the role of the supervisor when her supervisee recounts this excerpt from the work with a client? What issues can be identified that need addressing? How would the supervisor contract to work with this supervisee while she is seeing this client?

The following issues are important to bear in mind.

- The supervisor would want to consider the competence of the counsellor in their response to the excerpt from the client. If the counsellor was less experienced, the supervisor would be more concerned and more likely to intervene in the relationship; the supervisor would feel that the relationship between the counsellor and the client was being threatened by the client's behaviour which was described as acting out.
- The supervisor would need to be aware of the physical effects of the client's behaviour and be prepared to monitor this. If this is not done, does this attitude represent ethical and safe practice?
- The supervisor needs to maintain a balance between safety and control. This is a challenge to the supervisor who needs to ensure that the client is safe while simultaneously supporting the counsellor in her practice. The supervisee requires support as a person (the client's behaviour is affecting her, too!) and her competence as a counsellor needs to be maintained and supported. In how she handles this the supervisor models care and concern while not taking over and de-skilling the supervisee. This is an example of a parallel process being repeated from client and counsellor to supervisee and supervisor: empowering the counsellor while maintaining safe practice is an over-riding concern, and is repeated in the need to empower the client to get specialised treatment for the eating disorder.
- The supervisor needs to monitor the safety boundary. This client is potentially at risk: what is safe practice and how dangerous is the client's behaviour? What is the no-harm contract with the client, with the counselling organisation? What and how much support does the counsellor have from the counselling setting? This presents another parallel process in the supervision.
- The supervisor needs to clarify who has responsibility for the client work, who else is told of the client's behaviour and what are the limits of client confidentiality. Again this is a process which is paralleled in the counselling work.

- Who has the power? Discussion of this issue varies with the setting within which the counselling is taking place, the relationship between the supervisor and supervisee, between counsellor and client and the contract with the client. (This latter issue is more fully explored by Geoff Mothersole in 'Contracts and harmful behaviour', 1997.)

Conclusion

This chapter has highlighted some of the ethical and safety issues for supervision which emerge from counselling work with a client who abuses food as a metaphor for expressing feelings which are stirred up by the counselling process. It points out the importance that someone needs to assume responsibility for monitoring the client's eating and the subsequent behaviour, so that nutritionally as well as psychologically the client becomes healthy and does not jeopardise her life. The aim of the chapter is to leave supervisors with an increased awareness of the following issues.

1. The interface between physiological and psychological needs and the confusion created when food is used as a metaphor for feelings and abused as nutrition.
2. The links between ethics and safety.
3. The need to monitor who has responsibility for the physical as well as the psychological care of the client.
4. The boundary issue between avoiding or ignoring the eating behaviour and taking over responsibility from the supervisee in deciding how to proceed.
5. The importance of not becoming involved in arguments about body shape and weight, but interpreting the behaviour around food as a metaphor while ensuring that the client is learning about, or dealing with, food as nutrition elsewhere.

References

Bruch, H. (1979) *The Golden Cage.* New York: Vintage.

Krueger, D. (1989) *Body Self and Psychological Self.* New York: Brunner Mazel.

Mothersole, G. (1997) 'Contracts and harmful behaviour.' In C. Sills *Contracts in Counselling.* London: Sage.

Stern, D. (1985) *The Interpersonal World of the Infant.* New York: Basic Books.

PART 3

Issues in Integrative Supervision

Chapter 12

An Integrative Approach to 'Race' and Culture in Supervision

Maxine Dennis

Introduction

This chapter will highlight some of the issues involved in 'race' and cultural issues in supervision. After defining terms, an integrative approach to 'race' and culture will be suggested.

Henderson (Chapter 7) has used the terms 'deaf, dumb, and blind spots' regarding some elements of supervision. The saying 'familiarity breeds contempt' comes to mind in considering how topics have cycles of popularity and within these cycles the belief that, once examined, these anxiety-provoking topics can be laid to rest. All too often the sinking feeling of déjà vu, 'not this issue again' and 'we know all about this' raises its head when these topics are again discussed. Dennis (1998) noted that the American Association of Psychology, the British Association of Counselling (Codes of Ethics for Supervisors: BAC 1995) and the British Psychological Society Committee for Training in Clinical Psychology (1991) all recognised the need to integrate a multi-cultural perspective into clinical training in order to enhance the quality of therapy provided. The importance of this to the clinical and in turn the supervisory arena is self-evident. However, the impact of such integration in real terms is still a matter of debate.

This process (integrating multi-cultural perspectives in clinical training and supervision) has the potential to be creative but often ends up fraught and full of conflict with little, if any, growth or change occurring in more entrenched beliefs. There is often a tacit assumption that matching patient and therapist based on discernible characteristics like skin colour (ethnic matching) helps to deal with the complexity of ethnic and cultural areas. The supervisor who is black may help to support the black trainee in many ways, but specifically with feelings of isolation, provide a sense of acceptance and a role model that they can identify with less defensively. They can begin to challenge possible stereotypes and to integrate conflicting individual and professional identities.

While for some individuals 'matching' may be beneficial, the automatic assumption that this is always helpful cannot be made. Similarly, the paucity of supervisors who are black and from a minority ethnic group means that the choice of supervisor is limited. However, to elucidate the point: one counselling training course felt that a particular black trainee who was experiencing some difficulties could benefit from the support of a black supervisor. Needless to say, many of the difficulties were still evident with the new supervisor. Should supervisors go along with such arrangements? Is it in the interest of trainees, clients and training institutions? For the supervisor tackling the real issues or colluding with them is an ongoing struggle. In particular, this becomes evident when supervisors are commissioned to 'assess' and contain a 'difficult' trainee while avoiding the accusation of being racist. Their role in such an instance could be to prevent the institution being called racist.

Definition of cross-cultural supervision

Supervisors need to be aware of how 'race' and cultural issues are taught and indeed how they themselves have learned about these areas: messages are transmitted and translated across generations of therapists and embodied within the family of the professional institutions with which they are aligned. Whether the family of the institution enables its offspring to separate in a way that can produce new ideas and challenges to the institution or whether it simply maintains the status quo is a key question.

Particular aspects of the supervisory relationship are pertinent to all supervision but become more evident or exaggerated in cross-cultural supervision. There are different points of view about how race and culture respectively are conceptualised and whether they can be integrated within training or are taught separately. My own view is that both need to take place, that is integration within training as well as in a separate forum which is safe enough to contain anxiety. It is the capacity to think about the anxiety which the reality (internal and external) of racism arouses which is the source of hope and change (Cooper 1997) and one of the main foci of the chapter.

In defining cross-cultural supervision, Brown and Landrum-Brown (1995) suggest that cross-cultural supervision involves the contents, process and outcomes pertaining to the client, therapist or supervisory triad, in which at least one of the parties in the triadic relationship is culturally different from one or both of the other parties.

In order for those issues to be thought about within supervision the supervisor needs to have already begun the process of thinking about them. Much of the work has to occur within the supervisor to enable that process to take place in the supervisee. A supervisor needs to be aware of the supervisory focus: it is not helpful when colour consciousness becomes the sole focus of the interaction to the exclusion of other aspects, which may lead to over-identification with the oppressor.

Patricia Williams in the 1997 Reith Lectures gives a salutary example of colour blindness in relation to her son who resisted identifying colour and responded by saying it made no difference. As a result of Ms Williams's investigations this came to be seen as a social complication rather than a deficiency within him. It appears that the children in his class were told by a well-meaning teacher that colour made no difference, that it did not matter whether you are black or white, red or green or blue. Yet it did matter because the children were fighting over whether black people could play 'the good guys'. Williams states that the very confusion about colour constitutes an ideological confusion at best, and denial at its very worst. Equally important was that the teacher's dismissiveness left the individual (in this example her son) caught between what he experienced and the alienating terms by which social acceptance is sought. Neither colour blind, colour conscious or over-identification is helpful to the supervisory process.

A major pressure in teaching on 'race' and cultural issues is the desire to solve all ills. Therapy trainings vary in the degree to which 'race' and cultural areas are addressed, and supervisors often start from very different stances. Some people have a great deal of experience already in respect of race and culture and they view this as central to their work. For others an interest or desire to think in more depth about supervisory practice in relation to 'race' and cultural issues emerges slowly in their work.

Carter and Qureshi (1995) point to five different types of 'race' and culture teaching: the universal, the ubiquitous, the traditional (anthropological), the race-based and the pan-national. Briefly, they summarise these approaches as follows:

- from the universal perspective the focus is on human similarities and the therapist focuses on shared human experience
- in the ubiquitous approach multiple cultural identities are situationally defined and the therapist aims to be aware of difference
- in the traditional perspective culture and country are synonymous and race is seen as socially constructed and the use of exposure and cultural informants are central
- in the race-based approach the racial group transcends all other experiences. Culture becomes the value of such a group and those values, alongside the reactions of institutions in wider society, racism and racial identity is the focus for the trainee

- in the pan-national, culture is viewed globally but racial group membership determines one's place in the power distribution history and the psychology of oppression and domination in the therapy process.

From a supervisory perspective all these perspectives, with the exception of the universal one, are useful.

An integrative approach

An integrative approach to 'race' and cultural issues is a framework containing four key features: language, power, identity and institutional dynamics. These four features aim to transcend schools of thought and schools of counselling and supervision. Integrating a number of schools of thought may not attend to the issues, especially if those approaches are themselves oppressive. In thinking about an integrative approach the focus is less on integrating particular schools of thought than on integrating concepts. My own approach lies within an analytic framework using the dyad of the supervisor-supervisee relationship to examine the patient, the self-supervisee and the institution. All three relationships affect the patient, the supervisory relationship and the ability to contain the clinical work. Using the analytic approach the four areas can be considered.

1. Language

Language is dynamic and brings an uncertainty about which words to use. We need to examine the meaning of terminology and our associations with these terms. They are often used in a short-hand way but carry with them a historical and political loading that impacts on relationships in a multi-faceted way. They sometimes maintain rather than challenge the status quo.

Terms such as 'race' and ethnicity are all politically loaded, and especially heavily so in psychiatric settings (Sashidharan 1986). As Fernando (1988) states, culture is used in psychiatry in an ethnocentric way. Consequently, non-Western cultures that are alien to psychiatry are themselves seen as pathological. Thus 'culture' becomes the 'problem' that accounts for any abnormal behaviour of the client.

There is some debate about racisms (Phoenix 1999), that is the idea that 'race' affects different groups in different ways. It is meaningless to talk of racism as if it affected all in the same way. Others argue that the real issue of power and oppression is obscured by such a debate (Owusu-Bempah and Howitt 1999). It is clear that the black–white division is not the only story: Phoenix (1997), referring to Frankenberg (1993), states that 'race,' racism and ethnicity are also part of white people's lives, that is as a radicalised identity of white people. We cannot deny the impact of racism and capitalism, and the unquestioning acceptance of these by many whites as the norm (Phoenix 1987) along with the historical power relationships between black and white people (Hall 1992).

Culture includes the results of the behaviour of others, especially those who precede us. It is there which we begin life and contains values that are expressed and a language with which to express them. Culture contains a way of life that many follow, maybe unquestioningly, assuming there is not a better one. It includes language, music, art forms, preferences, appetites, aversions, rules, norms, standards, hopes, beliefs, attitudes, convictions and doubts, at least to the extent that these are shared, inculcated and transmitted from people to people. To be considered a part of a culture, anything, material or symbolic, need only to be of human origin, the man-made part of the environment (Segall *et al.* 1990; see also Fernando 1991 for definitions of race, culture and ethnicity). Racism is also maintained within systems by institutional racism defined as

> the collective failure of an organisation to provide an appropriate and professional service to people because of their colour, culture or ethnic origin. It can be seen or detected in the processes, attitudes and behaviour which amount to discrimination, ignorance, thoughtlessness and racist stereotyping which disadvantage minority, ethnic people. (Macpherson 1999)

2. Power

In many, if not all, instances the supervisor has the power to define the relationship: part of that power may be bestowed by supervisees who are in training. Even after qualification the supervisor is often more experienced, the one responsible for maintaining appropriate boundaries and so the power differential can be maintained. Some of these power complications are amplified when supervising across a cultural divide, when there may be a tacit assumption of what is defined as ordinary or normal. This relates to what we bring to supervision as supervisors and as supervisees, and which indirectly filters up from the patient. It also involves reference points that are assumed to be shared ones. It may seem obvious to check things out and be clear about this but such awareness may only become apparent with hindsight and not within the supervisory situation (Dennis 1999). Some questions worth considering are:

- how would you describe the culture of your supervision, that is the relationship you aim to establish with supervisees, and how is this connected to your traditions and the major influences on your life and thinking?
- what have been your experiences of good and bad supervision when you think of 'race', culture and ethnicity?

3. Identity development

The concept of identity development was first developed by Cross in the 1970s with reference to black identity and later applied to both white identity and those of mixed parentage. The underlying idea is that an individual moves through different stages of identity during their lifetime; this movement is not a linear one and earlier stages might be revisited depending on one's experiences. It is not without controversy, indeed the question of whether or not it exists is controversial (see Finn 1999; Owusu-Bempah and Howitt 1999; Phoenix 1999). This concept has been applied to supervision; a number of researchers have commented on it and it is clearly an area for further research. The original model was developed by Cook (1994), by Leong and Wagner (1994) for supervisees and by Priest (1994) for supervisors. In a review of the multi-cultural development of supervisor and supervisee, Carroll (1996) summarises the five main areas.

The supervisee's multi-cultural development is followed by the supervisor's multi-cultural development:

Stage One Unawareness: in this stage there is minimal awareness of ethnicity. The focus is on common humanity and therapy applies to all individuals; it is a colour-blind approach. In terms of the supervisor–supervisee relationship: 'I treat all trainees the same'.

Stage Two Beginning awareness: an awareness of discrepancies between cultures grows. The focus is on demographic and descriptive characteristics. There is recognition of cultural differences without actually knowing what to do with the information.

Stage Three Conscious awareness: the supervisee has conflicting emotions around cultural issues. They may be caught between their 'own' culture as normal and with struggling to apply theoretical orientations to other cultures. In the supervisor and supervisee relationship, it is represented by an attempt to identify differences and similarities between and amongst the respective cultures that make an impact on the supervisory relationship.

Stage Four Consolidated awareness: the supervisee has developed a multi-cultural identity. This stage represents the supervisor's attempts personally to discern where he or she fits into the overall cultural schemata.

Stage Five Transcendent awareness: the supervisee integrates personal cultural values, personal therapy and supervision values. At this stage the supervisor begins to appreciate cultural distinctiveness and identifies thought, process and communication patterns that facilitate supervision and assist the supervisee in learning therapy.

Stage six The supervisor is able to formulate multiple supervisory methodologies that are respectful of the supervisee's culture and interactive style while remaining professional in scope and nature.

4. Institutional dynamics

In each work setting there is a need to think about institutional dynamics and how they reverberate in the supervisory working relationship. Unless the managerial structure gives some credence to these issues (which are embedded in the very fabric of the institution) it can be difficult for individual work to have much impact. Similarly, in work with patients issues arise and impact the therapeutic relationship which may or may not be contained within the supervisory process. In supervision, as in clinical work, the issue of racism and institutional racism can have a pervasive grip. The following example gives some idea of how such organisational dynamics can impact supervisory work;

> A supervisee starts in a new setting having recently qualified as a counsellor. It is established on her first day that her past therapist is working in the same setting. Supervision is provided on a group basis but as the supervisee and therapist would be in the same setting there is a decision made to organise separate supervision for the supervisee. The supervisee has a succession of supervisors; they moved on due to promotions elsewhere. The supervisee has a new supervisor. At first there are a number of supervision sessions that are cancelled and when they eventually meet they discuss supervision and formulate a contract. The supervisory sessions seem to go well although there is some awareness of a slight weariness about the supervisee. The supervisee brings a succession of cases, usually black patients that are variously deprived and she thinks they have particular concerns about her being white and middle-class. As a supervisor you feel there is little evidence of that from the material brought. You are aware that from her work setting that the proportion of black patients brought to supervision far outweigh that of her case load. The supervisee is white English and older than the supervisor who is black and South Asian.

The key themes arising from this example revolve around how the supervisor tackles what seems to be an over-idealisation of all black clients and challenging whether alongside this apparent interest there is a deficient and denigrating image of blackness linked to the supervisor, which the supervisee contrasts with being white and middle-class. There is a need to unpack what the different terms mean, for example 'white and middle class', and the motivation behind their usage within the supervisory relationship. Also it is important to examine the relationship between supervisee and client.

Conclusion

Supervisors, as well as supervisees, are expected to participate in continued professional development with a cultural perspective throughout their working life. Such ongoing follow-up is helpful in enabling further development and a deepening of participants' understanding of the cultural perspective in supervision. This forms part of the recommendations contained in the BPS Continuing Professional Development (CPD) (1999) statement and the Daniels *et al.* (1998) *Briefing Paper of the Race and Culture Special Interest Group.* This may be more formal if working within the constraints of the health service and less so in private practice (as an institution or self).

Supervision needs to try not to overemphasise cultural diversity (Dennis 1999). Openness in thinking about the power dynamics between supervisor and supervisee enables both parties to name the unspoken and to feel less threatened by such a discussion. The supervisee may be more knowledgeable in this area than the supervisor. For example, a supervisee well versed in the Muslim faith or Judaism will know a lot more about the rituals and fine nuances of their religion and culture than those who do not share them. The supervisor can learn from the supervisee if they are secure enough in their position as supervisor. Supervisors can assess their own level of competence, foster a collaborative relationship and achieve a balance of inquiry without making the supervisee into the 'race' expert.

There is a need to identify early within the supervisory relationship with supervisees who are black or white what their thoughts are about 'race' and cultural issues. However, this is often seen as important only when one person in the relationship is someone who is deemed 'ethnic'. These issues can be lost from other supervisory triads or occur only as a clumsy after-thought when one is sufficiently guilt-laden to preclude creative thinking. These are not only issues for supervisees who are black, they are relevant to all. Such discussions need to be initiated irrespective of the cultural background of the supervisee.

Promotion of these issues within any institution is important and there is a need for structural changes which support individual work. For example within a reputable psychotherapy institution the first thing one encountered was the bust of a white king. The message conveyed was that this was head of the institution. The implications to the diverse community who came for psychotherapy were considerable. It took a lot of debate and thought for the bust to be removed and for the institution wholeheartedly to deal with the ramifications on both a conscious and an unconscious level. This is an example of the need to think about and question frameworks and practices which may prevent equal access. Issues about recruitment, environment and so on could also be usefully examined.

The assumption that supervisors are always 'white' needs to be challenged especially when this role reversal causes consternation within the supervisory relationship and therapeutically for some clients. Genuinely to integrate 'race' and culture issues in supervision and awareness of personal, professional and institutional cultures and their heritage is of primary importance for *all* supervisors.

References

BAC (1995) *Code of Ethics for Supervisors*. Rugby: British Association for Counselling.

BPS Committee for Training in Clinical Psychology (1991) *Criteria for Assessment of Postgraduate Training Courses*. Leicester: British Psychological Society.

BPS (1999) *Guidelines for Continuing Professional Development (CPD)*. Leicester: British Psychological Society.

BPS Standing Committee on Equal Opportunities (1994) *The Training of Clinical Psychologists*. Leicester: British Psychological Society.

Brown, M. T. and Landrum-Brown, J. (1995) 'Counselor supervision: cross-cultural perspectives.' In J. G. Ponterotto, J. M. Casas, L. A. Suzuki and C. M. Alexander (eds) *Handbook of Multi-Cultural Counseling*. Thousand Oaks, CA: Sage.

Carter, R. T. and Qureshi, A. (1995) 'A typology of philosophical assumptions in multicultural counselling training.' In J. C. Ponterotto, J. M. Casas, L. A. Suzuki and C. M. Alexander (eds) *Handbook of Multi-Cultural Counseling*. Thousand Oaks, CA: Sage.

Carroll, M. (1996) *Counselling Supervision: Theory, Skills and Practice*. London: Cassell.

Cook, D. A. (1994) 'Racial identity in supervision.' *Counselor Education and Supervision 34*, 132–139.

Cooper, A. (1997) 'Thinking the unthinkable: "white liberal" defences against understanding in anti-racist training.' *Journal of Social Work Practice 11*, 2, 127–137.

Cross, W. E. J. (1971) 'The Negro to Black conversion experience.' *Black World 20*, 13–17

Daniels, B., Dennis, M., Fatimilehin, I., Holland, S., Lokare, V., Nadirshaw, Z., Newland, J. and Patel, N. (1998) 'Services to black and minority ethnic people: a guide for commissioners of clinical psychology services.' *Briefing Paper Division of Clinical Psychology*. Leicester: British Psychological Society.

Dennis, M. (1998) 'Is there a place for diversity within supervision? An exploration of ethnic and cultural issues.' *Clinical Psychology Forum 118*, 24–32.

Dennis, M. (1999) 'Power and the supervisory process: the role of race and culture.' Conference paper given at Tavistock. London. Also available on tape from Tavistock Clinic Library, 120 Belsize Lane, London NW3 5BA.

Fernando, S. (1988) *Race and Culture in Psychiatry*. London: Croom Helm.

Fernando, S. (1991) *Mental Health, Race and Culture*. London: MacMillan Press.

Finn, G. (1999) 'Comparative visions and social identities.' *The Psychologist 12*, 3, 136–137.

Frankenberg, R. (1993) *White Women, Race Matters: The Social Construction of Whiteness*. London: Routledge.

Hall, C. (1992) *White, Male and Middle Class.* Cambridge: Polity.

Leong, F. T. L. and Wagner, N. S. (1994) 'Cross-cultural counselling supervision: what do we know? What do we need to know?' *Counsellor Education and Supervision 34,* 117–131.

Macpherson, W. (advised by Tom Cook, the Right Reverend Dr John Sentamu and Dr Richard Stone) (1999) *The Stephen Lawrence Inquiry: Report of an Inquiry.* London: HMSO.

Owusu-Bempah, K. and Howitt, D. (1999) 'Defective soul.' *The Psychologist 12,* 3, 138–139.

Phoenix, A. (1987) 'Theories of gender and black families.' In G. Weiner and M. Arnot (eds) *Gender under Scrutiny.* London: Hutchinson.

Phoenix, A. (1997) 'I'm white! So what? The construction of whiteness for young Londoners.' In M. Fine, L. Weis, L. C. Powell and L. Mungwong *Off-White Readings on Race, Power and Society.* New York: Routledge.

Phoenix, A. (1999) 'Multiple racisms.' *The Psychologist 12,* 3, 134–135.

Priest, R. (1994) 'Minority supervisor and majority supervisee: Another perspective of clinical reality.' *Counselor Education and Supervision 34,* 152–158

Sashidharan, S.P. (1986) 'Ideology and politics in transcultural psychiatry.' In J. Cox (ed) *Transcultural Psychiatry.* London: Croom Helm.

Segall, M., Dasen, P., Berry, J. and Poortinga, Y. (1990) *Human Behaviour in Global Perspective: An Introduction to Cross-Cultural Psychology.* Oxford: Pergamon.

Wiliams, P. J. (1997) *Seeing a Colour-blind Future: The Paradox of Race.* Reith Lecture. London: Virago.

Chapter 13

Anti-oppressive Practice in the Supervisory Relationship

Harbrinder Dhillon-Stevens

Introduction

This chapter will introduce, discuss and, I hope increase awareness on the theme of what is anti-oppressive practice and how it operates within the supervisory relationship. Clearly, the place to begin is the question: 'What is anti-oppressive practice?' Any answer to this question will need to tease out the differences between anti-racist, anti-discriminatory and anti-oppressive practice. Furthermore, the differences between culture, 'race' and ethnicity as concepts that are useful in understanding and working with anti-oppressive practice will need to be considered. The whole issue of anti-oppressive practice in the supervisory relationship requires tackling from both a theoretical and a clinical base.

Issues involved in anti-oppressive practice

Discussion on this theme usually raises more questions than answers. Often, the themes that emerge revolve around:

- power differentials, how to recognise and consider these at different levels between clients, supervisees, supervisors and institutions
- an acknowledgement or exploration of different frames of reference
- the need to be extremely questioning of ourselves and our own assumptions and being very patient and not punitive with supervisees who may be beginning to think about these issues
- formulating some basic principles that are not negotiable in the supervisory relationship, for example 'How can a supervisor be patient and tolerant with racist, sexist, homophobic ideas that a supervisee thinks are perfectly viable?'

- the importance of the contract and the working alliance at the onset of the supervisory relationship and making dealing with anti-oppressive practice very explicit within this
- struggling with 'How do supervisors operate in a way that is anti-oppressive while at the same time exerting appropriate authority as supervisors?'

In this chapter I am using the term 'black' to encompass people from Africa, Caribbean, Asia and ethnic groups who have a shared experience of racism. I recognise that not everyone will identify or share this definition.

Anti-oppressive practice

Counselling and psychotherapy often locate anti-oppressive issues within the 'cultural level'. Indeed, this is often where practitioners focus when considering issues between themselves and their clients or supervisees. This, I believe, leads to a multi-cultural approach which at present operates in terms of the phrase 'working with difference'. It is important to understand the re-emergence of this phrase from a political framework in the British context. It is due to this preoccupation with 'culture' in psychotherapy or counselling that supervisors or supervisees need to consider the difference between culture, 'race' and ethnicity. Fernando (1991) provides a helpful framework for exploring these differences. He noted how race and culture are frequently used as interchangeable terms. Furthermore, in defining culture one must look at one's own culture and values (the dominant culture) as this is often viewed as the 'norm' and used in judging other cultures in society.

Culture, I believe, is based on a number of factors such as: memories, ethnic identity, family attitudes to child rearing, class, money, religious or other celebrations, division of family roles according to gender and age. Cultures are neither superior nor inferior to each other.

Culture cannot and should not be thought of as static. There is a danger in the move to cultural awareness in the therapeutic relationship that cultural knowledge gained in working with one individual is applied to all individuals from that group rather than working with that individual in his or her cultural context. Dominelli (1988) refers to this willingness to learn about black people's cultures in order to practise culturally competently as the 'new racists'. Having cultural knowledge or awareness does not mean one is practising in an anti-racist and anti-discriminatory way.

'Race' is a socially constructed category to aid the justification of the systematic oppression of black people and create an ideology of racism. In this definition addressing positions of power is crucial in working with black or other marginalised groups. Racism is a belief that black people are inferior to white people in relation to their culture, religion, intellect, beliefs and lifestyles. It supports the belief that physical criteria determine intellectual and other abilities. It operates at individual and institutional levels.

In the British context, it could be argued that 'race' has been constructed in terms of being either 'black' or 'white'. Supervisors or therapists have been known to state that they do 'not notice the colour of clients' or ' I treat all clients the same, everyone is equal'. It would be interesting to research the impact of such comments on clients when their colour or their difference is not noticed. These statements are further compounded by the fact that society does not treat all human beings as the same. Comments such as these negate black people's experiences of racism and distance them from therapists. Clients may feel they cannot discuss issues of racism as the therapist will not understand, causing clients to internalise the racism in the therapeutic encounter. Furthermore, in the British construct, we need to pay attention to historical relationships between black and white people and how these still impact in the therapeutic space in terms of pre-transference (Curry 1964).

Ethnicity is another term used alongside race and culture. It is easy to forget that all people have ethnic origins, sometimes white supervisees or supervisors forget they have ethnicity and only use this concept in referring to 'black' clients.

Having considered the differences between culture, 'race' and ethnicity, supervisors and supervisees need to consider further the differences as well as the limitations in the concepts of equal opportunities, anti-racist and anti-discriminatory practice and anti-oppressive practice. Understanding these terms will be useful in practice as well as theory.

Equal opportunities

This concept is set in a legal framework, in the Race Relations Act 1976; the Sex Discrimination Act 1975; the Equal Pay Act 1970 and the Disability Discrimination Act 1995. The equal opportunities framework relates to the concept of discrimination and thus works to a model of challenging 'unfairness' and may be considered reformist in its outlook (Phillipson 1992). This means certain marginalised groups are already excluded from the equal opportunities dimension. The limitations of 'racial grounds' (Race Relations Act 1976) need to be considered alongside an awareness that there is no legislation that addresses issues of sexual orientation. People do not consider the limitations of this model and hence sometimes comment that they are working towards an equal opportunities policy or statement – this framework can often be viewed as paying 'lip service' to issues of anti-racist and anti-discriminatory practice and sustains the structures of oppression in our society.

Anti-racist and anti-discriminatory practice

Anti-racist practice is an approach that actively challenges racism and anti-discriminatory practice is an approach that actively challenges sexism, homophobia, ageism, ablism and other forms of discrimination. Both these approaches require supervisors or supervisees to be proactive in the therapeutic and supervisory relationship. However, these approaches are limited to the individual level as they require an active response of the supervisor or supervisee. In working with these dimensions, supervisors or supervisees need to ask 'What is it that I have to consider and do as a supervisor or supervisee?' Central to working in an anti-racist and anti-discriminatory way are the notions of responsibility and commitment and how we perceive our role as supervisors or supervisees.

Anti-oppressive practice

A model that works in terms of 'empowerment and liberation and requires a fundamental re-thinking and re-structuring of values, institutions and relationships' is that of Phillipson (1992, p.15). She suggests that, as practitioners, we need to think on a wider level than the individual level. To be aware of structural inequalities that exist in society and how systematic oppression operates in the lives of clients from marginalised groups is crucial to this model. Working at the individual as well as the structural level with clients is vital. For example, in working with a young Caribbean boy who had been attacked by three white youths, I held that we shared a common experience of racism but this may be perceived differently due to our different ethnic origins. Also, central to the therapeutic process was the issue of the Stephen Lawrence Inquiry and the boy's fears and experiences of how structural and institutional racism operate in British society and impact on him. I needed to understand both levels in order to engage fully with him.

Structural

The word 'structural' was used above and needs explanation. Structural is about considering social, economic, historical, political and cultural frameworks. Supervisors or therapists need to hold and work in these dimensions as well as at the individual level. However, it could be argued that all these dimensions are encompassed by the 'norm' or a white eurocentric framework. For example, people with disabilities may experience systematic oppression that able-bodied people do not experience. Supervisors or therapists can valuably question their experience and may own that in someone else's history or experience they may be oppressors for them. Acknowledging this, and naming it, conveys to clients that this dynamic is understood and responsibility will be taken for this at the individual and structural level. A psychotherapeutic process that does not take into account the person's whole life experiences, or that denies consideration of their 'race', culture, gender, sexuality or social values, can only fragment that person. It is easy to become stuck at the individual level because we feel ineffective and powerless at the structural levels. Hence, there is need to be clear from which frameworks supervisors or supervisees are working in the supervisory relationship.

Practice

What does all this mean for supervisors and supervisees in practice? A case scenario helps explore the principles of anti-oppressive practice in the supervisory relationship. The case example involves a black female supervisor and a white female supervisee: the supervisory relationship has existed for about four months.

The white female supervisee presents a client for supervision who is black and of mixed race parentage. The supervisee recounts an incident that occurred in her last session with the client that she wishes to explore. The client is talking about feeling something mysterious happening to her and struggling with this but keeps using the word 'mysterious'. The therapist interjects and states 'like voodoo'. The client becomes quiet, says nothing, leaves and does not attend her next session. The first response of the supervisee in relation to her intervention was 'I don't know where that came from'.

A number of areas are raised by this example:

- Does the supervisor need to make an anti-oppressive response as their first comment? Or is there a step before that? If this comment, made by the supervisee, was out of awareness then the supervisor making an anti-oppressive response may not help the supervisee. Does the supervisor need to raise this issue with the supervisee in terms of awareness? If someone does not bring something into awareness about my behaviour that may be oppressive, I am unlikely to consider or change my attitude, values and behaviour. How the supervisor begins the dialogue with the supervisee is crucial in providing a constructive framework in which to explore the issues.
- The supervisor may consider reviewing the working alliance between supervisor and supervisee and pay attention to the initial contract in terms of working within an anti-oppressive framework.
- Naming and discussing the power differences and imbalances between supervisor–supervisee not only in respect of roles, responsibilities, boundaries but in terms of race, gender, age, class, sexuality, disability might make for a further valuable intervention. How these may operate within the supervisory relationship, what each person's perception of these may be and how the supervisor–supervisee may contract in

dealing with these issues when they arise in the supervisory relationship or through ruptures needs to be considered.

A further point for consideration in the naming and discussing of power differentials is that some oppressions are 'visible' (race/gender) and some oppressions are 'invisible' (sexuality, class). In discussing 'visible' and 'invisible' oppressions the supervisor or supervisee needs to be aware that they have a choice about bringing invisible oppressions into the supervisory relationship while 'visible' oppressions are more explicit and may not offer supervisors, supervisees or clients a choice. Another important factor is that in discussing 'invisible' oppressions there may be very complicated and valid reasons for choosing not to disclose an 'invisible' oppression, such as sexuality.

Whatever the immediate intervention, what does seem important is that, in the contracting stage, it is essential to acknowledge the difference rather than the similarities between the supervisor–supervisee. In forging the working alliance there appears, at times, to be an investment in discussing the similarities in order to give the message that 'I can work with you' to the supervisee or client, rather than struggle with the differences.

With the supervisee in the case scenario, the issues raised in the first meeting by the supervisor were around race, ethnicity, gender, age and culture. The response from the supervisee were that these issues were not a problem from her perspective. The issues were left with the supervisor to re-name and re-frame in terms of a dialogue around them rather than them being a problem. The supervisor decided to start with the issue of age, experience and qualifications which were perhaps less of a threat to the supervisee and something with which she could easily identify. By naming these issues, even if they are not discussed in depth or with complete honesty (at this stage of the relationship), a platform is provided in the supervisory relationship to which they may be brought at some later stage. They have been acknowledged. This was an important factor in the supervisee bringing the issue and being concerned regarding her intervention, even though she did not fully comprehend the implications of her intervention.

Some supervisors prefer the word 'diversity' to the term 'different'. They feel that if they set up 'difference' they set up a barrier, but if they set up 'diversity' they set up the possibility of a conversation and 'dialogue'. Again, this raises the importance of language, and how there has been a shift in the arena of anti-oppressive practice to use the word 'diversity' as opposed to 'difference'. It is worth noting that the race and ethnicity of the practitioner influences the use of either term.

The notion of 'valuing difference' and 'frames of reference' and how these concepts related to the 'norm' in psychotherapy is a rich vein for discussion here. 'Valuing difference' in psychotherapy, is often a more comfortable approach for practitioners who are part of the norm (the dominant culture, in terms of race, ethnicity, ability, sexuality and so forth). However, what happens when one of the participants in the supervisory relationship is not part of the norm? Values come into operation around what is appropriate and from whose perspective. Psychotherapy, by and large, is located around the norm.

A further question brings up the impact of not acknowledging difference, for example, 'What might be the experience of a client or supervisee if a therapist or supervisor does not acknowledge there is a difference?' How might ignoring differences impact and reinforce the client or supervisee's experience and possibly give the message to the client or supervisee that these issues cannot be acknowledged, named and worked with or that they are not important in the therapeutic or supervisory relationship?

The difficulty with the term 'diversity' is that, often, the terms 'I work with diversity' have an undercurrent or unspoken message of 'I don't really have to look at my difference'. This is even more pertinent if the person is considered to belong to 'the norm' in society, for example white and able-bodied. It is easier to accept others' 'diversity' when one is of the norm and not challenged. Furthermore, the concept of 'diversity' and 'valuing difference' leads to power dynamics not being made explicit – they are ignored within these approaches. Occasionally, the question is raised about whether or not conflict is created by using the word 'difference' or whether the conflict is already there, that is, whether the supervisor can tolerate looking at the conflict and whether the supervisee feels they can work with a supervisor who can tolerate that conflict. Assumptions are rife here and the issue is whether these terms and concepts can be allowed, discussed, named and held in the supervisory relationship.

Going back to the case scenario above the use of the word 'voodoo' can be seen as a racist remark and the supervisee would need help in deconstructing the word and addressing how such a word may link to the client's systematic experience, how it perpetuates certain stereotypes of black people and its association with black people from a historical and cultural framework. Curry's (1964) concept of the pre-transference can help here. He describes this notion of the pre-transference as

> ideas, myths, jokes, fantasies and values ascribed to the black psychotherapist and his race which are held by the white patient long before the two meet ... the white client will have to work through this ... The white psychotherapist too will have to deal with this when working with black clients (Thomas 1992, p.137).

Therapists can not act with or alongside clients if they have not dealt with their own feelings raised about racism and its affect on their practice. The race of the therapist will affect the therapy.

Staying with the scenario it is worth exploring a number of further areas:

- How does the supervisee hear the black supervisor? If she has these attitudes and values towards the client what does she really feel towards the supervisor?
- When such ruptures do occur, one way forward is for the therapist to acknowledge that she has said something offensive, apologise and own her mistake. The taking of responsibility by the therapist (supervisee in this case) is central to a client staying in therapeutic contact and dialoguing with the supervisee. The client obviously felt unable to challenge the therapist's comments and this raised the question of 'What stage were the client or therapist in terms of their working alliance and therapeutic relationship? How had they contracted in terms of working together as a black client–white therapist?'
- It is important to remember that the supervisee did bring the incident to supervision and it needs to be seen in the context of a learning process. Following this incident the supervisee was able to bring further issues regarding anti-oppressive practice in her work. This is an indicator of self-reflection and a commitment by the supervisor–supervisee to dialogue and continuous learning in the supervisory relationship. Anti-oppressive practice develops over time and an accusing stance is not helpful. A learning stance for both supervisee-supervisor is more helpful.

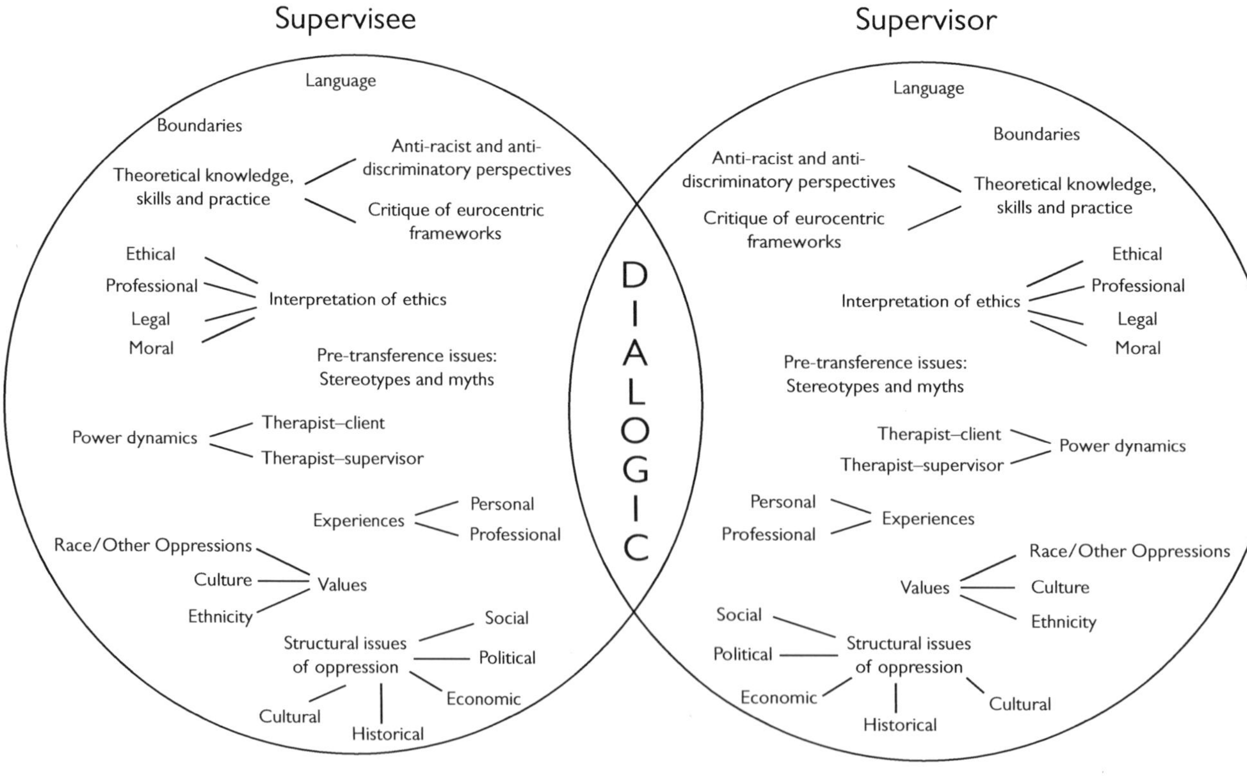

Figure 13.1: An Anti-oppressive approach to psychotherapy and supervision

Figure 13.1 is a model I have created and found useful in my work as a supervisor. This model encapsulates how issues of anti-oppressive practice occur in the supervisory relationship and how at different times these will be figure and ground for supervisor–supervisee. Furthermore, they can be seen as the 'basic principles' that need addressing in the initial meeting between supervisor–supervisee and for building a platform for dialogue in relation to anti-oppressive practice in the supervisory relationship.

Conclusion

This chapter highlights the struggles and complexities involved in working with anti-oppressive practice. My aim has been to highlight that anti-oppressive practice is an essential component for the growth, development and self-knowledge of the therapist supervisor and supervisee and is about good ethical professional psychotherapy and counselling practice.

References

Curry, A. (1964) 'Myths, transference and the black psychotherapist.' In J. Kareem and R. Littlewood (eds) *Inter-cultural Therapy.* Oxford: Blackwell.

Dominelli, L. (1988) *Anti-Racist Social Work.* London: Macmillan.

Fernando, S. (1991) *Mental Heath, Race and Culture.* London: Macmillan.

HMSO (1976) *Race Relations Act.* London: HMSO.

Phillipson, J. (1992) *Practising Equality – Men, Women and Social Work.* London: Central Council for Education and Training in Social Work.

Thomas, L. (1992) 'Racism and psychotherapy: working with racism in the consulting room: an analytical view.' In J. Kareem and R. Littlewood (eds) *Inter-cultural Therapy.* Oxford: Blackwell.

Chapter 14

Bolts from the Blue

Using Jungian Typology to Enhance Supervision

Charlotte Sills

Introduction

We are all familiar with those moments in therapy, counselling – or in life – when a feeling, a thought or an image seems to come to us out of nowhere. As psychotherapists we may call this an inspiration or an intuition, or we may analyse it as a response to a symbiotic invitation, or use concepts like countertransference or projective identification to explain it. In this chapter, I will use the Jungian theory of psychological types to offer a slightly different way of understanding those 'bolts from the blue'. Jungian typology will be described, followed by a method of using this theory in supervision (either of self or of a supervisee) in order to view these moments as important messages from the unconscious – not the whole truth but a significant piece of the jigsaw which must be gently brought into awareness.

The theory of psychological types

C.G. Jung (1971) identified four aspects of human functioning which he called sensing, intuiting, thinking and feeling. The first two functions concern people's way of perceiving themselves and the world and receiving information from it. The second two relate to how we make judgments and decisions about ourselves and the world. Everyone has the capacity to use all four functions but each of us has a preferred way of gathering information and a preferred way of organising it. In turn, of these preferred functions we are likely to have one function that is the strongest and most effective for us. It is known as our 'superior' function. We may then refer to ourselves as 'a sensation type', 'a thinking type' and so on.

One important point that comes out of the work is that we also have an 'inferior' or weak function, which will be the opposite of our strong one. Thus an intuitive type will be weak in sensing and vice versa. A feeling type will be weak in thinking and vice versa. Jung suggests that our weak function is lodged in our unconscious and will therefore be least under our own control. It follows therefore that it is this function which will provide the unexpected flashes of 'knowledge', the images or the hunches that seem to come to us like bolts from the blue.

This can be diagrammed, with the four functions grouped around a line representing the boundary between conscious and unconscious. Our superior function resides firmly in the conscious, our inferior one in the unconscious with the other two somewhere in between (at different times they could both be conscious, both unconscious or one of each). Obviously if a person has only one function fully in her conscious control, she will be restricted in her range of managing the world.

Feeling
conscious

Intuition

Sensing

unconscious
Thinking

Figure 14.1: A feeling type with intuition as the second strongest function

The four functions

Sensation types literally use their five senses (seeing, hearing, touching, tasting, smelling) to gather information and make sense of the world. This means that sensers attach high importance to tangible facts. They notice details and are excellent at working through problems in a pragmatic and logical way. Realistic and practical, they are normally very methodical and efficient though they may at times become somewhat overly concrete as their attention to facts may mean that they miss possibilities. They are grounded in the present and enjoy activities, often physical ones. When sensation is the inferior function, however, a person might suddenly notice a detail out of context which they erroneously take to represent a whole situation, or they might get a physical sensation or an image of an object.

Intuitive types tend to overlook details, even becoming impatient with them as they see the world in a broader way, absorbing a wide range of data and making sense of it as an impression of the whole. When seeing the following '...', sensers are more likely to see 'a row of dots' while intuitives may see 'a pause with something to follow'. Intuitives are especially different from sensers in that they are more interested in possibilities and new ideas for the future than they are in the realities of the present. Seeing patterns and connections between things, they are comfortable with change and good at initiating projects; they are exceptionally strong at knowing what should happen next. However, they are not so effective at carrying through a project in a systematic way, as the senser would do. When intuition is the inferior function, however, this ability to see connections and possibilities can become distorted, the person can experience unrealistic fantasies or become needlessly distrustful of the world.

The thinking type, as the name implies, likes to think things through carefully in a logical and objective way. While they do have emotions, they are likely to be able to put them on one side while they address a situation logically in order to work out what is the correct and fair solution. The thinker is rational, good at analysing and operates from clear and firm principles. He is good at understanding things, naming them and categorising them. He can sometimes appear rather unsympathetic as he deals with the facts and their consequences rather then how people feel or how they are affected. Thinking as an inferior function can produce the same capacity to name and categorise but this can be dismissive, negative or reductionistic.

Although the feeling type may be freer in showing emotions than the thinker, the word feeling in this case refers not to emotions but to a deeper experience of whether things 'feel right'. This means that they are likely to attach importance to subjective impression – both their own and others'. Feeling types are concerned with connection between people and are swayed in their judgments by how people feel in any situation. Their understanding of people is based on their empathy and ability to identify with others' feelings and circumstances. This empathic understanding inevitably springs from their own experience of life which leads them sometimes to believe that what 'feels true' (perhaps because it has been true in the past) must be the truth. They can sometimes, therefore, appear illogical to other people – particularly thinkers. When a person has feeling as an inferior function, he can be prone to flashes of feeling which he may not recognise so that they come out as irrational judgments. He is also likely to be the type of person who gets resentful and bears grudges.

The four types reflect their preferences in the way they communicate. Imagine four people going into a room and then later being asked to describe that room.

The senser may say 'The room is about 12 foot by 12 foot. It has two windows facing east. There is a bed in one corner, opposite a chest of drawers with a television on it. There are pictures and other decorations on the walls. On the other side of the room, there are two large chairs facing each other about five feet apart and a small, square table with a music deck on it. There are a lot of clothes on the floor and a slight smell of socks.' Notice the attention to facts and details.

The feeler may say 'It's a large room, full of clutter – clothes, papers, pictures, mess. The walls are pale grey, with dark grey velvet curtains. It is an impersonal room, even though it's full of signs of life. His clothes are everywhere, hundreds of tapes and so on. And the walls covered with pictures – photos of people and strange shapes. It has a nice big bed with a big duvet on it, covered in some dark material. It has chairs for sitting around but it's terribly untidy. It has nice high ceilings which make it light and spacious although it is too untidy really to enjoy.' Notice the attention to atmosphere and impression, the focus on colours, space and subjective response. The feeler has noticed that the room's occupant is a man but probably does not know how she knows.

The thinking type may say 'It's a bedroom, with seats for relaxing in. It is very untidy. There are a lot of clothes everywhere. There are jeans, trainers, shirts and the like as well as sports clothes and equipment. The room clearly belongs to a young man who plays sport. There are few books, and those visible are related to sports or are humorous, comic types so I assume that the person is not very academic in his interests. There are many photos on the wall – presumably of family and friends. The are also many pieces of artwork – drawings, models, and so on. They are not formally presented so are probably the work of the occupant'. Notice that, like the senser, the thinker pays attention to facts and details but in this case for the purpose of drawing conclusions, categorising, making sense of the contents of the room.

The intuitive type may say 'The room is part of an old house – probably used to be one of the main bedrooms. There's a blocked up chimney breast; if it were opened up it would make a really nice focus for sitting around. I wonder if the original fireplace was marble. It's got assorted furniture – probably passed on from some other room. If you put a sofa-bed in it instead of the bed, and got some interesting bits of furniture, it would make a fine bed sitting room. It's probably used for sitting around playing cards or chatting as well as sleeping. If the tree outside the window was trimmed back, it would have a view of the hills.' Notice the focus on links and connections, on possibilities and potential.

The reader may care to do this exercise for her or himself in order to get a personal sense of how the theory might work.

Jung, and his followers, developed the model to show the complexity of human beings. Nobody, of course, is purely one type. We are a unique blend of functions. Some of us are very strong in one or two functions and weak in the others. Some are only slightly stronger in one of the functions. In addition, what seems at first a clear division between types is complicated in therapy by the fact that the relationship between client and therapist or counsellor will have an effect on (both) people's presentation. We would describe a room differently if we were talking to our close and trusted friend over a coffee than we would to an estate agent. The other person's response would again affect how we continued the conversation. The same is true in the consulting room where the context and setting as well as the response of the therapist affects and influences the relationship. This is the co-creation of the field described by Gestaltists (Beaumont 1993)

An added subtlety is the effect of whether a person is an extrovert or an introvert. The extroversion–introversion polarity refers to our attitude towards life and whether our energy is put outwards towards the world and the people in it, or whether it is directed inwards in a more reflective way. Another way of considering this would be to say that the extrovert's point of reference is outside herself and the introvert's inside. The extrovert is energised by the outer world of people and things; he needs these outside referents in order to shape his own ideas. The introvert is energised by inner experience and needs to reflect carefully on his own in order to shape his ideas. A simple clue for differentiating the two in therapy or counselling is that extroverts stay in contact with their counsellor as they speak their minds or their hearts. Introverts need time to go inside and reflect before making contact to communicate with the counsellor.

The four functions in practice

It is evident, therefore, that a confident 'diagnosis' of a person's type configuration is subtle and complex. However, it is not essential, neither is it always possible for the therapist to be absolutely certain of the client's type or the supervisor of the supervisee's. This chapter simply hopes to alert the reader to the possibilities.

All four functions play an important part in therapeutic practice and in supervision. It may be useful to think about the various skills demonstrated by each function. Sensation involves, of course, the input of all the senses. The practitioner notices and observes, using what in Gestalt is called 'contact functions'. The therapist notices how the client sits, speaks, looks, smells. The supervisor notices all this about his supervisee and also inquires about the supervisee's client. How well has the therapist used his contact functions? What has he noticed? Under sensation we can also include collecting facts – how old is the client? What are his symptoms? What are his life circumstances?

The practitioner's intuition will tell him 'where the client has come from and where he is going to'. Intuition looks at the whole picture and sees a pattern emerge. Intuition is used in creating the 'ego image' (Berne 1961) and in holding a firm picture of the client's potential self. The intuitive function can also respond to supervisory questions like 'What will happen if this client goes on the way he is living now?' and 'What do you think needs to happen now?'

The thinking function is essential for making sense of the information. The practitioner gathers the facts from the client's past and present life and finds a way of conceptualising them. This is the arena of diagnosis and then treatment planning for the future. The thinking function is also the seat of understanding patterns and formulating interpretations.

Finally, the feeling function is the one that helps the counsellor make a real relationship with the client (or the supervisor with the supervisee). It is the function which seeks contact and makes it at the level of heart. It is also the function for empathic introspection, using past experience and 'how it feels' to understand the other.

In supervision, the supervisor consciously uses all her functions. She also invites the supervisee to use all his. In consciousness of Jung's model, the supervisor can observe the effects of the supervising process on the supervisee, monitor where it goes smoothly and seems relevant to the supervisee, notice if the supervisee responds with confidence or with tentativeness to suggestions for exploring the material or for treatment. She can direct questions towards the various areas such as 'What was happening at the time?', 'What do you think that means?' and so on, and she will notice that her supervisee responds with more facility to some areas than to others. Indeed, his 'stronger' functions may already have been apparent as he presented the client.

Being aware that people have different 'superior functions' can allow a supervisor to vary her interventions in order to help a supervisee use his strengths, develop his secondary functions and bring more of himself to the therapeutic encounter. For example, a supervisee presents something on which she would like some help. It might be a general question about a client or a concern over a particular session. The supervisor invites her simply to explore the issue by asking her questions, starting with the superior function and working 'downwards' to the inferior function. For example, a thinking type with auxiliary intuition may be asked: 'How do you understand this client's problems?'; 'What does this mean to you (or the client)?' (thinking); 'What do you imagine your client will do?' (intuition); 'What did you notice?' (sensation); and finally 'What does that feel like to you?' or 'How does she feel?' (feeling).

Bolts from the blue

It is not uncommon for practitioners to report having sudden flashes during a session, or for them to experience them during supervision as they are unfolding the material. These can be extraordinarily valuable contributions to the supervisory process. However, there are some caveats.

It seems that there are two ways in which counsellors, therapists and supervisors can make mistakes with these valuable messages from the unconscious. The first is to take the somewhat mystical view that the message must be 'the truth', simply because it seems to come from nowhere. The apparent magic of the occurrence and the feeling of 'knowing' that accompanies it invites us to suspend our critical faculties, and embrace the image, thought or feeling just as it is, assuming it to be a flash of intuition or a transpersonal phenomenon.

The second pitfall is to label it countertransference and, again, uncritically accept it as telling us some truth about the client. Commonly we assume that the experience is a result of projective identification (Ogden 1979) and actually belongs to the client. Or we may assume that it is some form of complementary countertransference (Novellino 1984; Racker 1968) and that we are being induced by the client's symbiotic invitation (Schiff and Schiff 1971) to respond to him in the way that, for instance, a parent figure did in the past. Both these ideas may indeed be true, but to call that the end of the story is to do our client a disservice.

I believe that these moments can be messages from our own unconscious; both disguised and lucid, both misleading and useful. Our unconscious can be enormously helpful to us, but it is also notoriously unreliable. It speaks in code, and can get things wrong. C.A. Meier (1995) writes:

> Jung felt he had proven that the inferior function is largely excluded from consciousness and thus exists in the sphere of the unconscious, where it can make its presence felt only indirectly and by means of rather peculiar effects. (p.13)

It is important to have a method of carefully exploring these 'peculiar effects' and bringing them fully into our awareness.

The method suggested here is for the person – either alone or with a supervisor or colleague – to identify the source of the message, in terms of function and then step by step, to bring her other functions to bear on the content of the 'bolt from the blue', starting with the function most close and gradually bringing the information 'up' into conscious awareness in order to plan treatment interventions and direction. In order to explain this method, a number of examples are given.

Jo, a supervisee whose superior function was intuition with secondary feeling was talking about her discomfort with a client. It was unusual for her and she did not understand it. Suddenly, with a shock, she said 'I keep thinking about the fact that he always pays cash, I've never seen his name written down anywhere. Maybe it's a false one, I know – I suddenly thought – he's a plant – he hasn't really come for therapy. He's here to spy – he's investigating something.' Jo is not given to suspiciousness, so it was very tempting to take this pronouncement as a flash of intuition. After all, one hears of journalists pretending to go for therapy in order to then write scurrilous articles in newspapers.

However, as this thought had come so suddenly, we knew therefore that it had erupted from the unconscious. Jo was firmly intuitive or feeling so that this hunch of hers must have been produced by her sensing function, abetted by her thinking. We began to explore what the message might have meant. Starting with her sensation function, we asked Jo what else she had noticed about her client which might be relevant. She said that her client had given few details about himself, and when Jo asked for them he seemed to avoid answering. He had a slightly supercilious air about him, and seemed a little critical. What was more, whenever Jo was empathic and understanding of the issues he discussed, he seemed to clam up and become evasive, implying that Jo had got it wrong. This was very strange as Jo is known for her empathic attunement. She began to reflect on the sessions – what did she do when her empathic understanding was avoided? She became even more empathic about his avoidance and asked more about the problem. What then? He suggested that it wasn't a problem really and changed the subject.

Jo was asked how she would diagnose her client using Paul Ware (1983). After thinking about his ways of viewing the world and general presentation and also using the 'feel' of him, she said 'paranoid'. We then discussed how a paranoid person might feel if the therapist was so understanding and empathic that she seemed to know more about them than she had been told. Jo began to understand that the more she 'knew' him, the more defensive he might feel. He may begin to wonder suspiciously how she knew these things, and indeed in some way if she was a spy or plant. Jo's bolt from the blue might indeed have been a concordant countertransference. She might be experiencing something of what her client did. Jo then used her feeling and intuition to work out what needed to happen in the therapy. She decided to be much less 'intrusive' with her empathy and spend more time working only with the material that the client brought.

Bob is thinking type with secondary sensation. In supervision, he described his work with a client who had been suicidal in the past. He suddenly said 'I feel frightened.' He was taken aback by his response and felt at a loss. He assumed it was an indication that his client was in danger. This was clearly his feeling function sending a message. It said much for his awareness that he was able to identify it clearly as a feeling. Starting with the nearest function to it – intuition – he was asked what he was frightened of, what might happen? At this point he surprised himself by saying that his fear was that he would make clumsy interventions and that his client would get annoyed with him and leave. Next, sensation function: what had he noticed in the sessions? He had noticed that he often had the impression that he was making mistakes. His client seemed dissatisfied with what he said or found small faults. Bob then used his thinking to make sense of what he was identifying. He realised that he had got into a 'Game' (Berne 1964) with his client and that he felt controlled. He also realised that this was reminiscent of the relationship he had had with his own mother. He was greatly relieved as he allowed himself to widen his view of what was going on in the therapeutic relationship and discuss his treatment plan.

Holly, a feeling type, was doing live supervision of a supervision session. It was the first time she had seen Harriet's work and she was not impressed. Looking at the trainee supervisor with some irritation, she suddenly thought 'Of course, she's a narcissistic personality.' This is a classic 'thinking function comment' of categorising and naming. It is also very typical of the sort of labelling that a feeling type can do as their thinking suddenly clicks in, which can make them sound sometimes rather opinionated and dismissive. The danger would have been for Holly to dismiss Harriet as someone who would never make a good supervisor. Catching herself in time, she referred to her second most inferior function – sensation. What had she noticed? She realised that she had seen Harriet confine her interventions exclusively to her own feelings and impressions and what she had noticed. Holly asked herself then what could happen (intuition). The supervisee had not been inquiring into her supervisee's experience nor that of the client. She needed to develop her range of interventions to ask how the therapist was or had been feeling, what her thinking was, how she conceptualised the client, what their relationship was like and so on. Holly's feeling function gave her a sense of how Harriet could be really effective with the right guidance. Accessing her thinking function again, this time under her own control, she thought of a supervision model that described several different areas of supervisory focus. She decided to give the article to Harriet so that she could reflect on it herself. In the mean time, having affirmed Harriet for what she had done well, she made two suggestions for different types of intervention. Harriet responded with interest and enthusiasm.

Readers are invited to experiment with exploring their own bolts from the blue by starting from the premise that a sudden flash of 'intuition' actually comes from our inferior function. It may manifest itself with 'peculiar effects'; in fact it often masquerades as its opposite, the superior function. For example, the thinking type assailed by a feeling of being threatened may make completely irrational statements, presenting felt values as reasoned facts. The feeling type may present as an expression of her feelings what is in fact a diatribe of name-calling.

The supervisor (or therapist) does not need to be sure of the person's typology in advance of using this method. It is enough to notice what is the nature of the 'flash'. Is it a feeling, a thought or categorisation, something that has been noticed or a hunch about something that will happen? That is likely to be the inferior function, which in turn gives a clue to the superior function. The work can proceed from there.

Conclusion

This chapter has focused on a method of 'unpacking' the bolts from the blue which are sent to us by our own unconscious mind. They can be enormously useful as a supervision tool and indeed a therapeutic one. Integrating them carefully into the rest of our functioning makes our use of these powerful flashes more reliable and more effective. There are many wider implications of the model for different areas of therapeutic work. For example, in relation to couples work there is potential for managing misunderstandings and miscommunications between different types. It is also possible (as Roy Ward suggested – personal communication) that some theories or approaches which are devised by and are particularly appealing to practitioners of one particular type may have a tendency to pathologise or ignore the strengths of the opposite type. There is the significant implication that supervisors may need to ensure that they are familiar with a range of different approaches in order to help their supervisees harness their strengths and develop their capacities.

Acknowledgements

This chapter contains an extract from Sills, C. and Wide, M. (1997) 'Contracts with different personality types.' In C. Sills (ed) *Contracts in Counselling.* London: Sage. It is reprinted here with the permission of the publisher.

References

Beaumont, H. (1993) 'Martin Buber's "I-Thou" and fragile self-organisation: Gestalt couples therapy.' *British Gestalt Journal 2*, 2, 85–95.

Berne, E. (1961) *Transactional Analysis in Psychotherapy.* New York: Grove Press.

Berne, E. (1964) *Games People Play.* New York: Grove Press.

Jung, C. G. (1971) *The Collected Works. Volume Six: Psychological Types.* London: Routledge and Keenan Paul.

Meier, C. A. (1995) *Personality. The Individuation Process in the Light of C.G. Jung's Typology.* Einsiedeln, Switzerland: Daimon.

Novellino, M. (1984) 'Self analysis of transference.' *Transactional Analysis Journal 149*, 10, 63–67.

Ogden, T. (1979) 'On projective identification.' *International Journal of Psychoanalysis 60*, 357–373.

Racker, H. (1968) *Transference and Countertransference.* London: Hogarth Press.

Schiff, A. and Schiff, J. L. (1971) 'Passivity.' *Transactional Analysis Journal 1*, 1, 71.

Ware, P. (1983) 'Personality adaptations: doors to therapy.' *Transactional Analysis Journal 13*, 1, 213–220.

Chapter 15

Which Sub-personality is Supervising Today?

John Towler

Introduction

The notion of the self being many selves, past and present, is well-documented in history, science, literature, theology and psychology. The idea that at times 'I am not myself' or that 'It was as if someone else was talking', is an indication that people have images of what Rowan (1990) calls 'the people inside of us', sub-personalities made evident in the work of Assagioli (1975) and Ferrucci (1982): 'One of the harmful illusions that can beguile us is probably the belief that we are indivisible, immutable, totally consistent being' (p.47).

The idea for this chapter arose out of my wish to produce a creative discussion about supervision as part of a training course. It will define the phenomenon of sub-personalities, and discuss through particular examples how some of my identified sub-personalities in the role of supervisor can impact on the effectiveness of the process of supervision. Sub-personalities, as ways of viewing self in the role of the supervisor or in the role of the therapist, need integrating into the whole person through the processes of identification, acceptance and integration (Whitmore 1991).

Defining sub-personalities

Rowan (1990) provides a masterly overview of the history of the idea of sub-personalities. He traces the idea, starting from primitive notions of altered states of consciousness and spirit possession (what he calls the 'stock-in-trade' of priests, witch doctors and shamans), through the changing social roles of the workplace, in literary characters like Hesse's 'Steppenwolf', in his own experience, and in the many psychological meanings afforded by the orientations of differing psychotherapies. He defines a sub-personality as 'a semi-permanent and semi-autonomous region of personality capable of acting as a person' (Rowan 1990, p.8).

Beahrs (1982), on the other hand, describes a sub-personality as a transitional state of being. Ferrucci (1982, p.47) uses images to clarify what he means by sub-personalities. He depicts them as 'psychological satellites, co-existing as a multiple of lives within the medium of our personality', and continues by quoting the poet Fernano Pessoa, 'In every corner of my soul, there is an altar to a different God' (p.47).

Rowan (1990) explains the phenomenon of sub-personalities in terms of disassociation along a continuum. At one end are the 'normal' transient states, for example mood swings which come and go with frequency; at the other, the state of multiple personalities which are ordinarily labelled as dissociated illnesses. The phenomenon to be considered in this paper is that state in between, that is associated with a normal state of being. In brief, from these authors, sub-personalities:

- exist
- are on a continuum between health and illness
- are able to be integrated into the personality as a whole to create
- are a person's potential for psychological healing and growth.

Identifying my own sub-personalities and exploring their impact on the process of supervision

I have become increasingly aware of particular sub-personalities in my role as supervisor. These have become increasingly evident in working with a group of counsellors from a company counselling service which has been undergoing major organisational change. I shall consider each sub-personality in turn and explore its impact on my supervision practice.

The crusader

What has precipitated my sub-personality 'crusader' or 'protector' is my need to defend the counsellors from being discounted by management. As a consequence, from time to time my anger at managers and the organisation has emerged in unhelpful ways, especially in conducting group supervision sessions.

One of the unhelpful consequences of this sub-personality is my collusion with the 'victim' position on the drama triangle (Karpman 1968) of the supervisee, that is, I find myself emotionally and cognitively wanting to distance myself from the managers and the organisation and to identify more closely with the supervisees. This is born of my intention to empathise with their pain and hurt at feeling discounted and unheard by their managers – to be like them. My own supervision has enabled me to face this tendency in myself and turn this collusion into an ability to become more psychologically distant from the supervisees. This enables me to recognise their victim position and to assist them to be potent in confronting that position.

My patterning is to please for fear of being disliked. My former chosen profession of priesthood encouraged me to be a rescuer and crusader, and the feeling that I am responsible for my flock twenty-four hours a day! I still carry elements of that past into my present supervision.

Does this need to rescue also come from a need to control – a form of narcissism? For example, do I know best? Again one of my temptations is to indulge in the formative function of supervision through what Heron (1991) calls 'seductive over-teach'. As a priest, teaching is also seen an important way of crusading.

Atlas

An associated sub-personality is that of 'Atlas'. Here I am seduced into feeling and acting that I am strong and invincible. 'Atlas' takes over when I feel that I am responsible for what is happening in the organisation and with the supervisees. At times I have found this a very intense feeling in supervision sessions. Let me recall an instance. A group of counsellors I am supervising have just been notified of radical changes which will impact on their practice and service to their clients. I am feeling sad, responsible and angry with the review body's projection on to the counsellors. This is expressed in an attack on the counsellors' apparent 'secrecy' regarding the confidentiality policy. I feel tearful in my empathy. The struggle to maintain psychological distance is immense. I find that self-disclosing about how I am feeling is an important way for me to maintain the distance, while remaining in touch with myself and with my supervisees.

Further reflection in my own supervision highlighted my feelings of being discounted, unheard, vulnerable and not strong.

H is an experienced counsellor. At the first group supervision following the announcement of radical changes to the organisation, he begins by saying how amazed he is at the reaction of a colleague who was so upset by the news that she went home for the afternoon: 'We need to get to grips with this'. I feel that he is attacking his colleague and me for my vulnerability. He needs me to be Atlas for him. I stop him twice. He challenges me. I reflect – what am I doing? At that moment in supervision I feel on the spot and accept the challenge. I'm not sure there and then what is happening. I accept that now he feels wobbly about expressing what was on his heart. I encourage him to continue with his perceptions about the changes. What follows happens with low energy. Clearly I have impacted on H's process, and the rest of the group are uncomfortable with the exchange. Their response is one of 'fence sitting'.

My subsequent reflections are as follows:

1. Was I in strong defending mode, protecting another supervisee who was not there to speak for herself?
2. Was I preventing H from expressing his projected fears about the current impact on him of the radical changes in the organisation? Was I not allowing him to feel weak?
3. My 'Atlas' sub-personality was active again in trying somehow to hold the organisation together. I felt I was responsible for what was happening. Maybe my attempt to rescue the absent supervisee turned into persecuting H for my perception of his judgmental attitude.

At a further supervision H and I explore what was happening between us. In reasserting his 'wobbliness' at my interventions, I am able to ask him to accept my vulnerability as a supervisor. By doing so I challenge my 'be perfect' driver (one of the sources of my Atlas sub-personality).

Where do these feelings come from? Why do I need 'to be perfect' and behave like Atlas? I guess I discovered early in my life that I found it difficult to get things right for my father. I was afraid of his anger and spent my time finding ways of pleasing him. I was strong because he needed me to be strong, I was young Atlas. If I didn't guess what he wanted and therefore get it right for him, then my fear was I would become the butt of his temper and that he would reject me. So is this the Atlas I am trying to be? I picked up the notion that I was responsible for meeting his needs. In retrospect it was a short step in choosing priesthood as a vocation and career. Here I took on the responsibility for so many people and what happened to them. As a direct consequence of this a realistic sense of my boundaries was frequently absent.

Mr Be-As-I-Am

I have another sub-personality who speaks to my Atlas. My therapy has been influential in creating my Mr Be-As-I-Am. On the face of it this might seem a sub-personality who has thrown in the towel – a fatalistic 'what will be will be'. He is allowing of others' choices and thus has no need to want to control. He is my authentic self, experienced and competent in the role of supervisor. Latently, he was always around in my mother. I trusted her and she trusted me.

Experiencing my break with the institutional church, the ending of my marriage and leaving my family, although unbearably painful, gave me an experience of internal chaos which cannot ordinarily be contrived. In the chaos I remember times of utter despair and emptiness combined with an intense feeling in my guts that somehow, somewhere I was OK. Friends came to my aid unbidden, my contact with my children continued and I found new work.

I believe this transition was seminal in the development of Mr Be-As-I-Am. I am reminded of Rogers' (1961) counsel 'trust the client', which comes from trusting self. Thus in my further dialogue with my supervisee H I allowed Mr Be-As-I-Am to be trusting and non-defensive, to own the unhelpfulness of my Atlas. I trusted that H was responsible for what he said and what he did. My world did not fall apart. He did not reject me. I did not need to get it right by pleasing him and exhausting myself by carrying the organisation and its pain on my shoulders. 'It is as it is, and I am as I am.' I believed that resolutions to the counsellor's dilemmas and the organisation's growing pains would be found. The signs looked hopeful. The dialogue between Atlas and Mr Be-As-I-Am continues. I feel a growing confidence in a healthy dialogue between them.

Sherlock Holmes and ardent listener

Sherlock Holmes has his roots in my Atlas sub-personality in that they share a common drive to be *all* embracing – my Atlas in being *all* responsible and my Sherlock Holmes in being *all* inquisitive! My Sherlock Holmes emerges in response to a supervisee's declaration of 'not knowing' and confusion about a client, combined with my innate curiosity about humankind. Another way of describing the function of my Sherlock Holmes is in his desire not to be found wanting, that is vulnerable in the face of 'not knowing'. I am comforted somewhat by the assertion of Bion cited by Casement (1985, p.4), 'In every consulting room there ought to be two rather frightened people; the patient and the psycho-analyst'.

One hypothesis of why he emerges so powerfully in some organisational settings is through the refractive phenomenon of 'parallel process' (Clarkson 1995). The confusion of the client is mirrored by the confusion of the counsellor in supervision. Instead of staying with 'not knowing' and the confusion of the supervisee, my Sherlock Holmes seduces me into searching for the missing information which will make it all crystal clear.

So where does my Sherlock Holmes originate in my psyche? My therapy has enabled me to understand more of the origins of my discomfort of 'not knowing', of finding ways forward and of resolution. My fear is that I will not be understood. Therefore, I need to demonstrate that I understand others so that they in turn will understand me. In my early childhood, I picked up the notion that I wasn't very intelligent and that I would have to strive hard if I were to make the grade. I wanted to be understood. If people could understand me, then I would know that I was intelligent. My small child felt he wasn't understood or even seen. I remember various early experiences in my family, school and church resulting in my carrying an image of this small, unintelligent, misunderstood boy into my adulthood. Somehow it was my fault. If I was not understood, the adults wouldn't bother to notice whether I existed or not. To inflict the same on others would be intolerable. My defence was to please others by putting myself out for people so that I would be noticed and somehow the possibility of being understood would be increased.

Living with chaos has been a challenge for me. I am aware how much initially I seek structure within groups and in other ways in my life. Becoming a priest was very attractive – a ready-made ordered life prescribed by form, ritual and providing answers to everything! An early marriage at 23 provided another prescribed structure to contain this need for certainty. At times as a supervisor when I experience 'not knowing' – a form of chaos – I feel small, inadequate, unintelligent and useless.

Sherlock Holmes as a helpful sub-personality promotes a healthy inquisitiveness into what is happening inside me, with my supervisee and the organisation (Lidmila 1997). He provides me with free attention, an ability to analyse, to assist supervisees to make sense of their experience by questioning the obvious.

Sherlock Holmes is unhelpful in times of pressure; for example, when I do not understand the supervisee's experience. At such times I make unhelpful interpretations or withdraw in anxiety. The following is an experience in organisational group supervision where I felt momentarily paralysed, totally inadequate and de-skilled as a result.

S, a supervisee, is a newcomer to the supervision group. From my first meeting with her I felt awkward. The organisation asked me to see her for an initial one-to-one meeting before the group supervision. I allowed myself to respond affirmatively to the organisation without thinking through the reasons for this. Why would I need to see her before the first group supervision? S felt I was hostile and unwelcoming as a result of our first meeting.

At the first group supervision S attended she was invited to say what she wanted and invited to contribute to a discussion about how the supervision was to be conducted. She said she didn't know, and only time would tell as to how useful it would be, and whether she would fit in. She spent her first working opportunity in the group reporting her work with her supervision group, and I felt excluded from making any interventions. I was aware of my ardent listener at work. At the end of the session there was a protracted discussion about times and dates for the next meeting. S asked that the time be changed. This was agreed by all the group members except one who said he would be on holiday.

At the next group S arrived one and a half hours late into the session which was scheduled to last for two and a half hours. She apologised for her late arrival. I said we needed to talk at some point about her lateness and future contracting with the group. She responded that she was an independent consultant and her commitment to the organisation for which she attended the supervision would need to fit in with her other work. She did not expect to be treated like a naughty child by a scolding parent. She had given up feeling guilty many years ago. Although she was paid for this contract in many respects she considered it as voluntary. T, another group member, then expressed how she felt she had not been heard and felt attacked by S. S said this was her projection. K, another member of the group, burst into tears, declaring that it was all too horrible, and please would S stop. H, another group member, reflected to me that he felt my introductory comment to S had an edge to it (passive aggressive?). S said she felt unwelcome, and that she didn't fit into the group. She said she was unwilling to share a reason for her lateness. T began to cry, and repeated how drained and exhausted she felt, and what was happening was not progressing attention to the clinical needs of her supervisees.

Initially, I felt paralysed. I felt I could not say anything to S without being misunderstood. I said I felt that whether she was paid or not I felt she needed to make a professional contract with the group that we all could understand and embrace. I felt I had let down the rest of the group. I felt that I was the cause of all this. However, I was able to draw the group to some conclusion within the time boundary by declaring my intention to work towards some resolution of my relationship with S.

On reflection I feel Sherlock Holmes in his compulsion to 'find out why' S was late was not up-front about how let down and irritated he felt, and my timing caused S to feel attacked. Certainly, Atlas was working overtime by the end of the session!

How did I manage a good enough resolution to this predicament? My Be-As-I-Am had a calming effect on me towards the end of the session which allowed me to sit back, take deep breaths, and make a statement to S and the group. Mr Be-As-I-Am recognised his companion ardent listener who listened attentively but did not feel the need to continue with a sterile discussion, nor to continue to make unhelpful interpretations, nor needed to understand there and then. Ardent listener said to Sherlock Holmes: 'After you have listened to the best of your ability right now, you may "know" some more, or not; you have the right to stay with your listening and respond when you feel it is appropriate and helpful. What you say is your truth: you may differ from another's but that is what you have to start with.'

Ferrucci says that by not accepting a sub-personality, we cause its involution; that is its potential to cause complications. We need to treat sub-personalities with understanding in order for them to open up and give us the best of themselves. In understanding my Crusader/Rescuer sub-personality I am noticing my sub-personality's polarity, that is my ability to respond to the request of the supervisee acknowledging my own limitations in a sense of 'we-ness'. In using my Crusader/Rescuer sub-personality I am hooked into a distorted domain, better described as my Atlas sub-personality. Here, I assume a God-like quality in imagining and acting as if I am omniscient and omnipotent. In utilising my Sherlock Holmes I need to temper his inquisitiveness by listening to my Mr Be-As-I-Am. My internal supervisor counsels me to:

1. Be respectful and give reflective time to understand my sub-personality.
2. Allow my sub-personality's polarity free rein.
3. Raise the sub-personality to its highest potential 'and discover that every psychological aspect has in itself the seed of its own transformation' (Ferucci 1990, p.58).

Conclusion

What this chapter has enabled me to do is to begin to process my effectiveness as a supervisor through:

- identifying some of my own sub-personalities
- recognising their strengths and weaknesses
- accepting their impact on my being and on my supervisees
- working with them to integrate them into the whole of me
- creating the possibility of dialogue between my sub-personalities
- living with the tension which exists between them.

While I have identified but a few of my sub-personalities, I recognise that the field for discovery and identifying others is limitless.

Stone and Winkelman (1985), like Ferrucci, give timely warning about what happens when I choose not to face a particular sub-personality because of its potential unpalatability: 'The energy pattern we disown turns against us' (Rowan 1990, p.69).

Watkins (1986), a Jungian analyst, encourages me in this imaginal work when she writes, 'Personifying is not an activity symptomatic of the primitivity of mind, but is expressive of its dramatic and poetic nature' (p.58).

Which sub-personality is supervising today? While my inclination is to want a synthesis of my different selves, my reality is that they remain being themselves in their variety, richness and colourfulness all capable of dialoguing with each other. I am the one and the many. They are who I am and who I may be.

References

Assagioli, R. (1975) *Psychosynthesis: A Manual of Principles and Techniques.* London: Turnstone Press.

Beahrs, J. O. (1982) *Unity and Multiplicity: Multilevel Consciousness of Self in Hypnosis, Psychiatric Disorder and Mental Health.* New York: Brunner/Mazel.

Casement, P. (1985) *On Learning From the Patient.* Tavistock: Routledge.

Clarkson, P. (1995) *The Therapeutic Relationship in Psychoanalysis, Counselling Psychology and Psychotherapy.* London: Whurr.

Ferrucci, P. (1990) *What We May Be: The Visions and Technigues of Psychosynthesis.* Aquarian: Thorsons.

Heron, J. (1991) *Helping the Client: A Creative Practical Guide.* London: Sage.

Karpman, S. (1968) 'Fairy tales and script drama analysis.' *Transactional Analysis Bulletin 7,* 26, 39–43.

Lidmila, A. (1997) 'Shame knowledge and modes of enquiry in supervision.' In G. Shipton (ed) *Supervision of Psychotherapy and Counselling: Making a Place to Think.* Buckinghamshire: Open Uuniversity Press.

Rogers, C. (1961) *On Becoming a Person.* London: Constable.

Rowan, J. (1990) *Sub-personalities: The People Inside Us.* London: Routledge.

Stone, H. and Winkelman, S. (1985) *Embracing our Selves.* Marinadel Rey, CA: Devorss and Co.

Watkins, M. (1986) *Invisible Guests: The Development of Imaginal Dialogues.* Hillsdale, NJ: The Analytic Press.

Whitmore, D. (1991) *Psychosynthesis Counselling in Action.* London: Sage.

Chapter 16

Supervision
Researching Therapeutic Practice

Martin Milton

Introduction

Several personal issues provide the background to this chapter. First is my interest in the relationship of theory and research to practice in therapy and supervision. This relationship came into focus for me through both of my professional posts and my own areas of study. One of my posts is as a trainer on a doctoral training in counselling psychology where the model of the scientist–practitioner is adopted, and the second position is as a clinician in an NHS department of psychology. In this second setting the NHS and governmental forces related to 'evidence-based' practice is an essential guide. My efforts to complete my doctorate also had me thinking a great deal about the relationship between research and practice. Why was I doing this research if it would be completely unrelated to my practice as a therapist? Surely there was some link?

Integrative approaches to supervision (the title of this book) focus on different models and approaches to supervision and how supervision is perceived and carried out by senior practitioners in the field. Attention is also given to the integration of individual and contextual factors into practice – especially issues relating to where and how individuals live, work and practise. This chapter has a slightly different focus as it explores the dilemmas of the supervisors who actively want to integrate science and practice, research and therapy.

Supervisors and research

Supervisors' relationship with research is frequently ambivalent. Some possibilities could include their hope to:

- 'update' their thinking regarding research
- seek ways in which research might validate therapeutic and supervisory roles in work contexts
- consider the degree to which supervision might legitimately be seen as a research process in itself
- explore the gap between the practice and academic worlds
- find a research topic
- consider whether supervision can re-search the self of the supervisee. In this respect, the supervisor need to acknowledge and consider the gender biases that affect practitioners' ability to undertake research, use it, or get it published.

Research is also associated with difficult emotions such as shame, guilt and indifference for many practitioners. This is not exclusively the case though; some may feel that their excitement about research and the recognition that they have some strengths should not be overlooked, although this could easily happen in systems where research is given a low priority.

Brief review of the literature

The literature appears to be characterised by three different approaches.

1. The first is reflective in nature, with authors reflecting on their own experience (Mearns 1991; Milton and Ashley 1998; Moore 1991). These accounts provide descriptions of the supervisee's and supervisor's aims for supervision and their experiences of the processes of supervision.
2. The second is concerned with the development of a number of models of supervision (Carroll 1996; Hawkins and Shohet 1989; Page and Woskett 1994). This literature attempts to define the tasks of the supervisor and the supervisee and how these can be effectively undertaken.
3. There is also a literature that addresses supervision from a model of therapy. These authors address two main areas. One is the skills needed and the processes that occur when supervising a particular model of therapy. There are also some papers that address the application of particular therapeutic principles and theories to the task and processes of supervision and these are addressed by representatives of a number of schools, for example existential (van Deurzen-Smith and Spinelli 1996; Pett 1995; Wright 1996), psychodynamic (Langs 1994), client centred (Frankland 1993, unpublished dissertation; Patterson 1982),

Gestalt (Muntz 1983) and rational emotive behaviour therapy (Wessler and Ellis 1982).

The literature is not characterised by clarity or consensus, even about the usefulness of supervision (Holloway and Neustedter 1995) and this may be related to the fact that research might validate the work of supervisors and the role supervision has to play in the therapeutic enterprise. This lack of clarity is an issue as the therapeutic professions frequently deem themselves to be scientist–practitioners. There is a literature on the scientist–practitioner model of practice.

Supervisors may note that many texts still remind us that there is a gap between research and practice, with academics being accused of producing research that is not useful to the practitioner and accusations that practitioners are unaware of important research (McLeod 1994; Roth and Fonagy 1997). This gap is problematic as many contexts demand that we evaluate our practice, for example how the NHS values evidence-based practice and many professional guidelines.

What supervisors think of research

As there are many forms and functions of research it is important to clarify what is understood by the term 'research'. Some possibilities are listed here:

- the polarity between the qualitative or quantitative paradigms with difficulties in the use of both
- the view that research 'is all about numbers and columns' and aims for conclusive evidence
- research is about making assumptions explicit
- alternatively research is about disproving or questioning what is assumed. It pays to be curious
- research can also be experienced as too big a project to undertake, with too many variables to consider.

Some of the questions a researching supervisor ought to bear in mind are:

- who is the research ultimately for?
- who will benefit from the results?
- do research methodologies match the language or process of therapeutic or supervisory practice?
- when supervisors think about actually undertaking research, it is important to identify the dimensions being researched; is it a small study, using oneself and one's clients? Or does it need to be more

extensive and call upon colleagues and/or particular groups of supervisees or clients?

- how does one find the right question? Clarifying this enables the project to be manageable, offers access to participants or garners support from funders or managers.

Research and scientific discourse

When considering the issues above, it is important to relate the issues to the literature and accepted models of research practice available to those involved in supervision and the therapeutic professions.

1. There is a traditional formal academic research often based on positivist, quantitative methodologies. This approach is evident in random control trials (RCTs) on the efficacy of different forms of therapy. This type of research often evokes anxiety on two levels: first, about the relevance to supervisory and therapeutic practice; and second, about the participants' own ability to understand or undertake such research.
2. There are also studies on the outcome and process of therapy, or research that explores a particular phenomenon, for example the role of expressed emotion in the families of schizophrenics. Research in this tradition may be useful for practitioners to be aware of and to be consumers of. This would mean that it is important for supervisors to be aware of this literature when helping those that ask about research in supervision.
3. There is another form of research, which is more qualitative in nature, and is embodied in such approaches as thematic content analysis, narrative, conversation or discourse analyses, grounded theory and feminist research. Supervisors can also recognise that case study methods and the presentation of verbatim notes in supervision are related to these methods. This is important when considering the qualitative paradigm and the desire for research methods to match the nature of supervision and therapeutic practice.

All these different types of research may have a place in a cycle of research. Supervisors need to develop understandings of a phenomenon, check their understandings in relation to the phenomenon being explored, look to see whether their understandings are as accurate as they think they are, and the like. While involved in this process they are undertaking research. There are of course other aspects of the research cycle including hypothesis generation and dissemination of findings which would carry this process into the wider world.

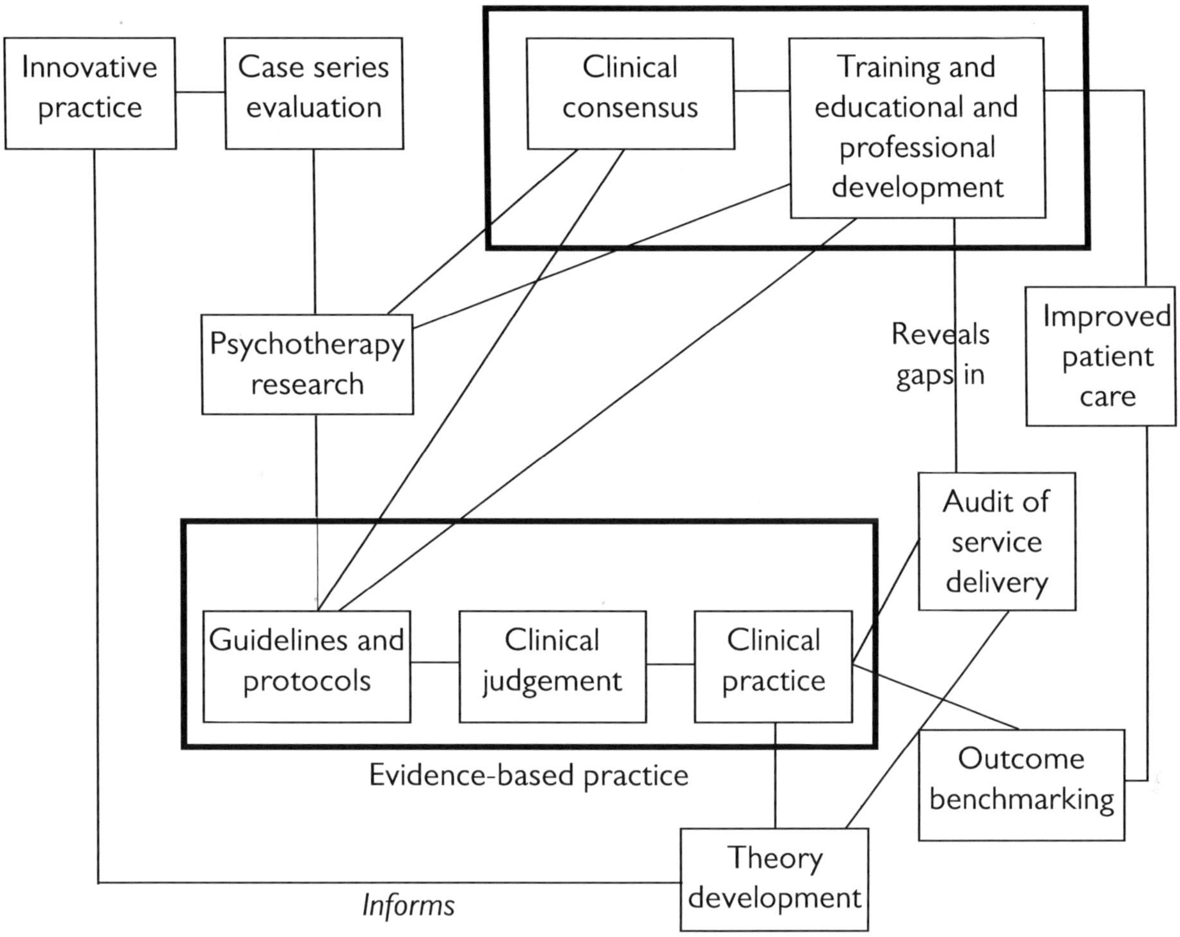

Figure 16.1: Professional consensus. From NHS Executive (1996)

The diagram in Figure 16.1 was originally published in the NHS Psychotherapy Services in England: Review of Strategic Policy (1996), which is a government sponsored review.

This model can be thought to privilege some views over others, for example the traditional view of science and the cognitive behavioural approach to psychotherapy. In line with this, can some models of psychotherapy and counselling to be included or validated by research be seen in this way? This view of science and research can be difficult to marry with the experience and values of supervision and therapy, and the concept of processes set in black and white flow diagrams and figures contrary to supervisory beliefs.

It also raises some interesting questions about the role of research and the power it is given. For instance, does the evidence of the efficacy of one model (such as cognitive behaviour therapy's efficacy with the emotional disorders) disprove the role of person centred therapy? While this may be the impression gained from medical and other discourses it is an error of logic. As outlined by Roth and Fonagy (1997), while there is evidence to support the use of cognitive behaviour therapy, there are difficulties that mean that psychodynamic, systemic (and other approaches) are less easily slotted into this way of viewing science. What is difficult is to quantify relational factors, or to research them 'objectively'.

What is the role of therapeutic supervision in this model? The professions state that supervision is crucial to practice. Employers pay a lot of money for it (or in private practice, therapists fund the expense themselves), yet there is no formal evidence (Holloway and Neustedter 1995) that supervision actually helps the client.

But is not supervision a form of applied research in itself? Supervisors and supervisees have hypotheses about clients, they ask questions about them, collect information (data) and then think about it (data analysis). The supervisee (or at times the supervisor) may write the 're-search' up in case studies or more frequently in letters to referrers. There is frequently a hope that the 'findings' will influence those who might find it useful, primarily the client but also the therapist's own development, and others that may be related to the client, for

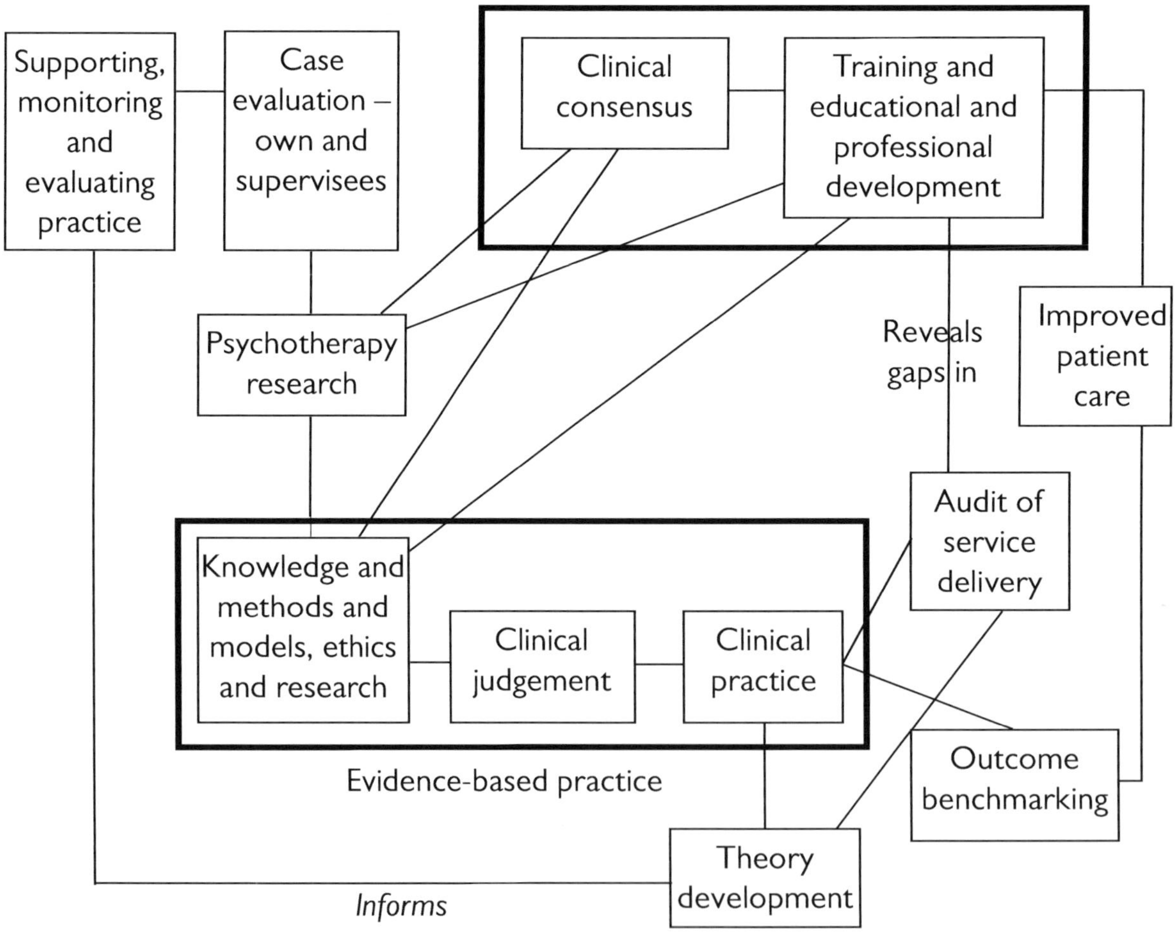

Figure 16.2: Professional consensus. Original from NHS Executive (1996); adapted in the light of participants' considerations

example the referrer. Where supervision fits into the research cycle can be summarised in Figure 16.2, an adaptation of the original.

When seen in this way, the above detailed diagram and the ideas of evidence-based practice easily marry with the supervision process, although of course this needs to occur with a respect for other forms of knowing other than causal knowledge. The guidelines and protocols available to supervisors parallel knowledge of a range of models of practice that supervisors frequently bring to their work as senior members of their professions. An awareness of what is ethical practice is also relevant here. These domains of information are useful in the evaluative function of supervision, which could be related to the need to audit service delivery.

Case series evaluation is an area that supervisors are privy to by virtue of their own clinical work and that of their supervisees. Another idea is that as they are not able to completely 'manualise' human interactions, the therapist is always at the level of individually tailored therapy, thus always being engaged in a form of innovative practice. At least some of the time, supervisory efforts take the form of advising on a formal attempt to research practice, for example the writing of a case study and so on. However, it also takes the form of using methods akin to qualitative research methods to elaborate and consider the phenomenon that the client brings as requiring attention.

Reflections: considering supervision in relation to research

How can supervisors become more comfortable in using existing research skills more or how can they begin to develop research skills, if they had been lost to any degree? To evaluate this, supervisors can focus on the following three questions.

1. What do you feel are your current research skills and how do they help or hinder your practice as a therapy supervisor? Supervisors need to remember that they are skilled at 'widening out' phenomena, 'focusing in' and clarifying meanings and processes. They also consider how the core values implicit in supervision are useful in allowing supervisees to feel safe and therefore be open and honest in their considerations.

2. What would you need, by way of research training or updating, to feel confident about more formally exploring or evaluating aspects of supervision or therapy practice? Supervision training could provide 'more research training'. In relation to this, employers might be asked to provide such research updating as a form of CPD. 'Time for theory and practice' could be considered in work time rather than in supervisors' and supervisees' own time. It is important that supervisors and research be 'taken seriously', and in this regard the idea of a 'separate supervision journal' is a possibility. It seems that appropriate fora are

again a research issue, and the dissemination of research findings a crucial aspect of the research process. Clarity over where this information can be located is important for both those undertaking it and those who want to use it.

3. In view of the alleged gap between research and practice, between academics and clinicians, consider your view on this and consider how such a gap might be bridged. There is indeed a gap between research and practice, but this is narrowing because of the increased academic components of training, both therapy and supervision training.

Conclusion

While I previously felt that ethical practice and the contexts of the health service required us to consider, both as therapists and supervisors, the issues that have come to be conceptualised by the term 'evidence-based practice', this chapter has helped clarify my own thinking. This is not a clarity where I feel that I have all the answers or evidence at my finger-tips, rather a recognition that it is important to have an evaluative eye in our every day work. Indeed, I share many of the hopes and confusions, anxieties and quandaries of my colleagues. By creating a dialogue with colleagues, supervisors can become clearer on how they might begin actively to seek for answers (and to some extent the questions too).

The position supervisors occupy by the demands of the professions, alongside people's pain and distress, requires them constantly to consider the impact of their theories and their practice. While they may not have a clear idea of 'what works for whom?' (Roth and Fonagy 1997), and maybe never will, it is still important to think about their work and examine the evidence for supervisory decisions and actions. Without such a focus they run the risk of being no more than bound by blind faith and in doing so may unintentionally add to the confusion and distress that they engage with as therapists and supervisors every day.

References

Carroll, M. (1996) *Counselling Supervision: Theory, Skills and Practice.* London: Cassell.

Deurzen-Smith, E. van and Spinelli, E. (1996) *Two Different Aspects of Supervision in the Existential-Phenomenological Approach to Psychotherapy.* Video distributed by MindSearch Enterprises.

Hawkins, P. and Shohet, R. (1989) *Supervision in the Helping Professions.* Milton Keynes: Open University Press.

Holloway, E. and Neustedter, S. (1995) 'Supervision: its contributions to treatment efficacy.' *Journal of Consulting and Clinical Psychology 63*, 2, 207–213.

Langs, R. (1994) *Doing Supervision and Being Supervised.* London: Karnac Books.

McLeod, J. (1994) *Doing Counselling Research.* London: Sage.

Mearns, D. (1991) 'On being a supervisor.' In W. Dryden and B. Thorne (eds) *Training and Supervision for Counselling in Action.* London: Sage.

Milton, M. and Ashley, S. (1998) 'Personal accounts of supervision: phenomenological reflections on efficacy.' *Counselling 9*, 4, 311–314.

Moore, J. (1991) 'On being a supervisee.' In W. Dryden and B. Thorne (eds) *Training and Supervision for Counselling in Action.* London: Sage.

Muntz, E. (1983) 'Gestalt approaches to supervision.' *Gestalt Journal 6*, 1.

NHS Executive (1996) *NHS Psychotherapy Services in England: Review of Strategic Policy.* Leeds: NHS Executive.

Page, V. and Wosket, S. (1994) *Supervising the Counsellor: A Cyclical Model.* London: Routledge.

Patterson, C. H. (1982) 'A client-centred approach to supervision.' *The Counseling Psychologist 11.*

Pett, J. (1995) 'A personal approach to existential supervision.' *Journal of the Society for Existential Analysis 6*, 2.

Roth, A. and Fonagy, P. (1997) *What Works for Whom: A Review of the Psychotherapy Research.* London: Guilford Press.

Wessler, R. L. and Ellis, A. (1982) 'Supervision in counselling: rational emotive therapy.' *The Counseling Psychologist 11.*

Wright, R. (1996) 'Another personal approach to existential supervision.' *Journal of the Society for Existential Analysis 7*, 1.

Chapter 17

How Supervisors can Protect Themselves from Complaints and Litigation

Gary Leonard and Joanna Beazley Richards

Introduction

In general, supervision for counsellors takes the following forms:

- independently purchased supervision dealing with counselling issues
- line management supervision of employed counsellors
- a hybrid situation where an employed counsellor is supervised by his or her line manager but also has counselling supervision brought in from an independent supervisor.

Before proceeding further, it may be appropriate at this point to define what is meant by complaints and litigation. Briefly, by complaints we mean formal complaints concerning the conduct of a counsellor or supervisor which are dealt with by their employer, professional body or other organization, but does not include litigation before the civil and criminal courts. Litigation involves proceedings being instituted against a counsellor or supervisor before the civil courts (county court or high court) or criminal courts (magistrates court or crown court).

Complaints and litigation

Complaints may be made in a number of ways and have varying degrees of seriousness. Examples of the types of complaints that a supervisor may have to consider are as follows:

- a direct complaint by a client to a counsellor
- a direct complaint by a client to the counsellor's supervisor or employer

- a complaint by a client to the counsellor or supervisor's professional body
- a complaint to the Police concerning the conduct of the counsellor and/or supervisor.

It has to be said that the circumstances in which a supervisor could be the subject of a complaint to the Police as a result of conduct on the part of the counsellor are likely to be rare. These types of complaints are however also likely to be the most serious and potentially to have the most far reaching effect. It is therefore important that these complaints are given serious consideration and dealt with effectively at an early stage.

Complaints may be made in isolation or in conjunction with litigation instigated either by the complainant in the civil courts or by the Police in the criminal courts. For example, a client who alleges that he or she has suffered harm as a result of inadequate counselling and supervision of the counsellor may complain to the professional body governing the counsellor and the supervisor. The client may also institute civil proceedings in the county court or high court against the counsellor and supervisor. In general terms, all but the most serious civil claims are dealt with before the county court. Subject to certain exceptions, a claim has to have a potential value of £50,000 before it can be dealt with before the high court.

A client may also complain of improper conduct on the part of a counsellor which constitutes a criminal offence (a sexual assault, for example). This may lead to a complaint to the professional body of the counsellor and supervisor as well as a complaint to the Police in relation to the conduct of the counsellor. It is fair to say that the supervisor is unlikely to have any criminal liability in such circumstances unless or he or she participated in the criminal offence. It is however appropriate for supervisors to be aware of this danger and to be on their guard.

No one involved in any sort of dealings with the public can wholly insulate themselves from complaints. People will make complaints, with or without justification and counsellors and their supervisors, like all professionals, must be prepared to deal with them quickly and effectively. Similarly, it is not generally possible to block litigation against a counsellor or supervisor in advance. It is however possible to lay the foundations of a strong defence by ensuring that adequate records are kept which will help rebut any allegations made by the person bringing the claim.

One of the best strategies for dealing with complaints and litigation is to try to avoid creating a situation where the complaints can arise in the first place. This is best achieved by ensuring that the client knows exactly where he or she stands with the supervisor and that proper notes of all dealings with the client are kept by the counsellor.

From the supervisor's point of view, it is important to ensure that counsellors are dealing with their clients in an ethical and business-like manner, that adequate notes are being kept and that there is a proper agreement detailing the scope of the relationship between the counsellor and the client.

Legal liability

The same rules apply in general terms for avoiding liability in the field of litigation. It is worth being aware however of the bases upon which counsellors and their supervisors can be sued. This helps provide a perspective upon any threatened or actually instituted litigation.

Legal liability can arise in a number of ways. As far as supervisors are concerned however, their liability is likely only to occur in relation to actions carried out by counsellors in the ordinary course of their work. For example, a supervisor may have some liability in relation to continued unethical conduct towards a client which arises as a result of inadequate supervision. A supervisor is, however, unlikely to be held responsible in the event that a counsellor acted wholly out of character on one occasion and, for example, struck a client.

A supervisor's legal liability to a client is governed by the Law of Torts. In simple terms, in order to establish liability against the supervisor, a client would have to establish that the supervisor owed him or her (the client) a duty of care. He or she would also have to show that the supervisor breached the duty of care and that as a result the client has suffered some loss or damage.

It is important to note at this point that there are three issues here: first, the duty of care; second, the breach of the duty of care; and, third, loss or damage following on from the breach. The absence of one or more of these elements will be fatal to a claim against the supervisor. For example, it would be difficult for a supervisor to argue that he or she did not owe a duty of care to the clients who were seen by a counsellor in the ordinary course of the counsellor's work which was under the supervision of the supervisor. The situation however would be considerably altered if the counsellor saw someone outside the usual scope of their practice without the knowledge of the supervisor. This might arise where a counsellor provides help to a friend without bringing that work within the scope of his or her practice and without making any notes which would come to the attention of the supervisor.

The second element of any claim requires there to be a link between any breach of the duty of care on the part of the supervisor and the loss suffered by the client. An example of this might arise where a supervisor had concerns over a period of time (perhaps three months) as to the standard of counselling being provided by the counsellor. If the supervisor did not intervene adequately during that period and the client suffered harm, it is arguable that the client could successfully claim that the supervisor had breached his or her duty of care. If however it could be shown that the harm was not in any way affected by the supervision, it is likely that the client could not establish liability on the part of the supervisor. An example of this might occur where the counselling had taken place and the client had suffered some arguable harm prior to the routine supervision. In such a case, the supervisor could not have had any input into the case and would not have had any opportunity to discharge his or her duty of care.

Finally, it is important to note that in each case of a claim for damages against a supervisor, the client must show that he or she has suffered loss or damage as a result of the supervisor's actions. If a supervisor has been lax in supervising the counsellor but this has had no direct affect upon the client in that the client has not suffered any harm or loss, no compensation will be payable.

It is perhaps worth mentioning in passing that a potential liability may arise where only the counsellor is being sued but the counsellor chooses in turn to bring proceedings against the supervisor, alleging inadequate supervision. This could be done either by joining the supervisor to the existing proceedings brought by the client or by the counsellor suing the supervisor for breach of contract.

Examples of this are as follows:

Example 1 Smith is providing counselling services for Jones. Smith is a self-employed counsellor who buys in supervision from White. Smith's counselling is inadequate and White fails to pick this up during routine supervision. As a result, Jones' condition deteriorates and he sues Smith. Smith feels that the problem is at least partly attributable to the lack of supervision from White and therefore applies for White to be joined to the proceedings so that the court can assess the extent to which Smith and White are liable, if at all, towards Jones. If the court found that they were equally liable, each would pay half of the compensation to Jones.

Example 2 As in the example above, Smith is providing counselling services to Jones under the bought-in-supervision of White. Once more, the services are inadequate and Jones suffers harm. Once more, Jones sues Smith. In this case however Smith does not bring White into the proceedings but defends them himself. At the end of the proceedings, an award of damages is made against Smith. Smith then takes separate proceedings against White alleging inadequate supervision and breach of contract. Part of the compensation that he claims is the cost of the damages that he has had to pay to Jones. Jones is not involved in the proceedings between Smith and White.

Let us look firstly at the position of the independent supervisor whose expertise is bought in by a counsellor or other organization providing counselling services. In this type of case, the best way of avoiding liability is to ensure that the scope of the supervisory relationship is properly documented and that adequate notes are kept of the supervisor's dealings with the counsellor. In the absence of any clear link between the client and the supervisor, or evidence that the supervisor was put on notice of the client's predicament, it is unlikely that an independent supervisor could be liable for any misconduct on the part of the counsellor.

It is worth noting that where a supervisor is put on notice of an existing or potential problem relating to the relationship between the counsellor and the client, the supervisor may in those circumstances bear some liability for any harm suffered by the client if he or she fails to intervene adequately during the supervision process. For example, if it became apparent to the supervisor, either from a discussion of the case with the counsellor or as a result of direct contact from the client, that there was a serious problem with the advice being given so as to put the supervisor on notice of potential harm to the client, the supervisor could in most circumstances potentially share liability for the misconduct of the counsellor.

Where such a serious problem arises, it is suggested that the only effective way of dealing with it is to give written advice to the counsellor as to how the supervisor considers the matter ought to be handled, with the proviso that the supervisor will withdraw from supervision if his or her advice is not followed by the counsellor. This should be coupled with a timetable for any remedial action required and the supervisor should ensure that these communications are all recorded in writing and that he or she is prepared to withdraw from supervision if the advice is not followed.

It may be said that these guidelines for supervisors are easier to outline that they are to put into action. Indeed, this is a fair comment. One way of ensuring that the guidelines are followed as much as possible is to require any supervised counsellor to enter into a binding contract with the supervisor which sets out the records that the supervisor expects the counsellor to keep and the type of agreement that the supervisor requires the counsellor to enter into with his or her (the counsellor's) clients. The supervisor would of course have to check on the existence of the notes and the contracts regularly as part of the supervision process. This would help to ensure that basic standards were being maintained.

In the case of an employed counsellor, it is unlikely that his or her line manager or employer could escape liability for any negligent actions as they would not be in a position to distance themselves from the counsellor's conduct in the same way as an independent supervisor. The only way for a supervisor or employer to protect themselves from the consequences of the misconduct of an employed counsellor is to ensure that the supervision is sufficiently rigid and thorough so as to prevent, so far as possible, any potential liability arising in the first place.

The employer or supervisor of an employed counsellor will not be liable for any acts committed by the counsellor which are outside the usual scope of his or her employment. Thus, as mentioned above, the employer is unlikely to escape liability where the client suffers harm as a result of clearly inadequate counselling. This is in fact likely to be the case whatever the standard of supervision. If, however, the counsellor starts seeing the client outside of the work environment and the client suffers harm as a result of events beyond the knowledge of the employer, such as the breakdown of a relationship between the counsellor and the client, the employer could in those circumstances argue quite convincingly that the harm suffered by the client was totally outside the scope of the employer's business and there should therefore be no liability on the part of the employer.

It should be noted that the liability of a supervisor will be much the same, whether the supervision is paid or unpaid. The liability really arises from the existence of a duty of care and not as a result of the financial arrangement between the supervisor and counsellor.

Conclusion

The points made above have addressed in general terms the potential liability that a supervisor may have as a result of complaints or legal proceedings brought against him or her by a client of the counsellor. It is also worth considering in passing the potential third party liability that may arise from this relationship. This refers to any harm suffered from someone who is not actually involved in the counselling process but who suffers as a result of the actions or lack of action on the part of the counsellor. For example, a client may disclose an intention seriously to harm a third party. Where a supervisor is put on notice of such a threat, he or she may have some liability towards that third party if inadequate guidance is given to the counsellor in relation to the risk and the third party as a result suffers some harm.

To protect themselves in relation to potential complaints and litigation, we want to emphasise that supervisors should:

- know their relevant codes of ethics and professional practice and abide by them
- have regular supervision on their supervision work
- keep detailed records of the supervision they give, and the outcome of supervision they receive, including the scope of all contracts and agreements and the terms and conditions applying.

Epilogue

Supervision in the Millennium

Brigid Proctor

Introduction

Where does supervision presently stand in relation to our professional associations of counselling and psychotherapy? At present, there is a lack of systematic integration of supervisor training and practice into any kinds of professional bodies. This needs to be considered not just theoretically as a good idea but looking also at the 'who' and 'how' as well as the 'what'.

There is disturbingly little communication between supervisor trainers and supervisors in the field, with each other and with professional bodies in counselling and psychotherapy.

How can we begin to establish proper channels:

- between supervisors
- between those who train supervisors
- between trainers, supervisors and professional associations?

The challenge is to set up, service and maintain much needed

- systematic support and challenge for supervisors and supervisor trainers
- systematic channels for gathering information and validating the effectiveness and ineffectiveness of counselling and psychotherapy
- systematic integration of supervision and supervision training into professional systems, associations and so on.

How else can we be a self-monitoring profession based on the universal requirement for ongoing supervision?

Where are we now?

A list of what systematic channels of communication are available to supervisors and supervisor trainers and between them and professional associations includes the following:

- British Association for Supervision Practice and Research (BASPR)
- Codes of Ethics and Practice for supervisors
- Accreditation procedures for supervisors
- considerable new literature in the field of supervision
- debate in most counselling and psychotherapy journals on supervision
- supervision as an accepted requirement for practitioners and trainees
- informal groups to discuss and debate supervision issues
- a formal network of psychodynamic supervisors
- new research within supervision from MSc and doctoral courses
- a new sub-editor in charge of supervision for the BAC journal, Counselling.

In addition to the above there was a position paper on supervision, instigated by BAC, which pointed out the lack of support and communication for supervisors within BAC and which suggested some concrete recommendations. Chief among these was that BAC should:

- encourage meetings between supervisor trainers to identify common needs and practice in training supervisors with a view to formulating a 'core curriculum'
- clarify the extent of 'clinical responsibility' within supervision
- clarify the recommendation of 'supervision' for counsellors against whom complaints were found
- facilitate some forum for regular meeting of supervisors
- institute channels of communication between any forum and professional committees of BAC
- actively encourage research in supervision.

It is still not clear what will happen in response to this paper since new committees have been in formation within BAC.

What do we need as supervisors, how can needs be met and who will take responsibility for meeting them?

One possible way ahead is to focus more on the role of BASPR so that it might become a more formal association in its own right; publish its proceedings (less cheaply than in book form); be bigger and more accessible; invite workshops openly; and establish a formal link with BAC. How feasible is this?

An earlier organisation SCATS, (Standing Conference for the Advancement of Training and Supervision), that met annually experienced the difficulty (indeed lack of success in that case) of making a shift from conference to association, and the time, energy and funds needed.

The pros and cons of supervisors moving from being part of the counselling and psychotherapy 'profession' to a body or profession in their own right is worth mentioning. The challenge concerns who would be active in creating any forum – within or outside other associations. Connected to this is the fact that supervisors are also counsellors and very often have other roles – trainer, manager, committee member and so on, and that the time and energy available for focusing regularly on supervision issues is therefore limited.

Other ways ahead include:

- more information being given to the general public about supervision (but what should be said when we know so little about what supervisors are being trained in and what they actually offer?)
- supervisors being required to have training
- training courses for supervisors being accredited or having some regulation and comparability
- a supervision journal, or space dedicated to supervision within other journals
- more research on supervision
- groups or networks of supervisors meeting regularly to exchange ideas and practice
- creating an e-mail mailbase for supervision.

Conclusion

Supervisors *are* their professional associations. What is worth doing to promote the importance of supervision to the effectiveness and credibility of the practice of counselling and psychotherapy depends on someone taking initiatives and being prepared to devote time to follow them through. This is most likely to happen if supervisors meet regularly with colleagues more frequently than once a year. That way, initiatives and resulting work could be shared.

Postscripts

Since the conference, Jane Speedy has set up a mailbase for supervisors and circulated the address to everyone who was at the conference (mailbase@ mailbase.ac.uk).

The BAC (now BACP) Journal *Counselling* is to come out ten times a year (instead of four) and will have an assistant editor responsible for a regular supervision section.

Contributors

Rita Arundale is married with two adult children and enjoys singing, dancing and reading as well as eating out and foreign holidays (preferably at the same time). After many years in administration, during which time she began studying at The Northern Guild for Psychotherapy, Rita made a career change in 1994 to become a full-time counsellor and supervisor, working in a variety of settings but mainly in primary care. She has an MSc in Counselling in Primary Care as well as a diploma in humanistic counselling and a certificate in supervision. She trained for four years as a psychotherapist in transactional analysis before deciding not to follow that route. She is currently studying to gain a diploma in supervision.

Joanna Beazley Richards, M.Lit, MSc, BA(Hons), Cert. ED, Dip. TMHA, CPsychol, TSTA, AFBPS, FRSM, MBIM, is a freelance chartered psychologist with clinical and forensic specialties. She is also a UKCP registered psychotherapist and teaching and supervising transactional analyst. She is founder and principal of Wealden College of Counselling and Psychotherapy, which offers fully accredited training for these professions. She is a registered expert witness and founding member of the Institute of Expert Witnesses. She has a particular interest in the legal issues associated with the practice of counselling and psychotherapy and with supervision. She has over 30 years experience in this field.

Michael Carroll, MA, PhD, is a Fellow of the British Association for Counselling, a Chartered Counselling Psychologist, an Associate Fellow of the British Psychological Society and a BACP Accredited Supervisor. He works as a counsellor, supervisor, trainer and consultant to organisations in both the public and private sectors specialising in the area of employee well-being. He has published widely, particularly in the areas of workplace counselling and counselling supervision.

Graham Curtis Jenkins worked as a general practitioner paediatrician in the National Health Service for 28 years. He became the first director of The Counselling in Primary Care Trust in 1991 which was set up to promote, support and develop counselling and psychotherapy in general practice in the UK. He is the author of many research papers, book chapters and reports on child care, mental health and counselling in primary health care.

Maxine Dennis is a clinical psychologist working in psychotherapy with adults in London. She has a long-standing interest in the teaching and integrating of 'race' and cultural issues within clinical psychology training. In addition she is also concerned with the provision of culturally-appropriate psychology and psychotherapy services. Currently chair of the BPS 'Race' and Culture Special Interest Group, she has published widely on training and supervision issues for clinical psychologists.

Harbrinder Dhillon-Stevens is a UKCP registered integrative psychotherapist and has an MSc in integrative psychotherapy. She also holds a BA (Hons.) in politics, a certificate of qualification in social work (CQSW) and has been senior lecturer on the postgraduate diploma/MSc in social work at South Bank University for the past nine years (part-time). Harbrinder also holds a diploma in supervision and is a qualified Institute of Training and Development (ITD) trainer. She is a primary tutor on the MSc integrative psychotherapy at the Metanoia Institute and also works as a child art psychotherapist, having undertaken her training at Guys and St. Thomas's Medical and Dental School, University of London. She has a private practice and undertakes therapeutic work with children, young people and families.

Dagmar Edwards, MSc, Dip. Couns., Dip. GPTI, UKCP registered psychotherapist, Accredited Trainer of the British Association for Counselling and Psychotherapy (BACP), has trained in a range of approaches to therapeutic work, including person centred, Gestalt, transactional analysis and systemic family psychotherapy. Formerly head of the person centred counselling course at the Metanoia Institute, she has many years' experience in the development of clinicians, both as a trainer and a supervisor. She also has over ten years' experience as a manager in a large organisation and has had considerable involvement in the implementation of change programmes within the organisational setting and in the training and facilitation of work based groups. Dagmar is a director of Psychology Matters and has a private practice in counselling, psychotherapy and supervision, and in clinical and organisational training.

Penny Henderson, BA, Msc, Dip. Coun., works independently. An accredited counsellor, she offers counselling, supervision of counsellors, organisational consultancy, training about communication and teamwork and team building for organisations. She is also an associate of the Counselling in Primary Care Trust and contributes to the training of medical students in Cambridge.

Julie Hewson, BA (Hons.), Cert. Ed, Dip SW, CQSW, TSTA, CTA, BAC registered supervisor and former assessor of supervisors, Registered with UKCP. Julie is director of the Iron Mill Centre in Devon and Cornwall providing counselling, psychotherapy and supervision training as well as management consultancy services. She has delivered supervision training in the Czech Republic and currently works in Dublin and Zurich. She is completing her PhD in the area of shame in supervision.

Gary Leonard is a Southampton solicitor and founding partner in Leonard and Swain solicitors, a firm specialising in litigation, including professional negligence and civil liberties issues. He and his firm have been involved in professional negligence litigation and complaints procedures involving a wide range of professionals, including doctors, psychiatrists, counsellors, nurses, social workers, accountants, surveyors and other lawyers. A member of the Law Society's Children Panel, he has nearly 20 years' experience of child care cases and related issues.

Martin Milton, DPsych., is a chartered counselling psychologist and a UKCP registered psychotherapist. He is joint course director of the University of Surrey Doctorate in Psychotherapeutic and Counselling Psychology. He is also attached to the South West London and St. George's Mental Health NHS Trust.

Vanja Orlans, MA, MSc, MSc, PhD, Dip. GPTI, ATSM (GPTI), AFBPsS, UKCP registered psychotherapist, chartered occupational psychologist and chartered counselling psychologist, has extensive training and experience in a range of approaches to therapeutic work, as well as in the understanding of group and organisational dynamics, and has been working with individuals and groups in many different settings for over 20 years. She is a supervisor for several training programmes in London for both counsellors and psychotherapists and is also an examiner for a number of programmes concerned with clinical training, both in the UK and abroad. She has published articles concerned especially with organisational stress and related issues, and has had considerable involvement in the implementation of counselling within work settings. Vanja is a director of Psychology Matters, and has a private practice in counselling, psychotherapy and supervision, and in training and organisational consulting.

Steve Page is Head of Student Support Services at the University of Hull, where he was previously Head of the Counselling Service. A BACP senior registered practitioner, he has a background in private practice and theraputic communities. Steve is also involved in training, research and writing. He is author of *The Shaddow and the Counsellor* (Routledge 1999) and co-author (with Val Wosket) of *Supervising the Counsellor* (Routledge 2001)

Brigid Proctor, since retiring as the director of counselling courses at South West London College in 1987 has worked as a freelance counsellor, supervisor and as consultant to supervisors, trainers and counsellors. She is also a trainer and writer. Formerly a member of the BAC Executive and first convenor/chair of both the standards and ethics and training sub-committees of BAC, she is now a BACP fellow as well as an accredited supervisor. She supervises counsellors working in a variety of statutory, voluntary and business organisations. She is author of *Group Supervision: A Guide to Creative Practice* (Sage 2000).

Jane Rosoman qualified as a psychiatric social worker and worked in child psychiatry. She trained at the Tavistock Clinic, specialising in systemic psychotherapy and consultation. Subsequently she was involved in counsellor training and development through the Westminster Pastoral Foundation and the University of Surrey at Roehampton. Clinical supervision within organisational settings and consultation to organisations are a major part of her professional practice. Her approach is integrative and she is particularly interested in therapeutic interventions in primary care systems where she has experience going back over twenty years.

Charlotte Sills, MA, MSc, PGCE, Dip Syst. Int. Psych., UKCP registered psychotherapist is a counsellor and psychotherapist in private practice and has worked as a trainer and consultant in a variety of settings. She is a qualified transactional analysis clinician and a teaching and supervising transactional analyst. She is author of a number of publications on counselling and psychotherapy. Charlotte is head of the Transactional Analysis Department at Metanoia Institute in West London.

Jane Speedy is a lecturer in the Graduate School of Education, University of Bristol. She has particular interests in the field of counselling at work, adult education principles in counselling education and research methods in counselling training and supervision.

Margaret Tholstrup, MSc, is a chartered counselling psychologist, an associate fellow of the British Psychological Society, a UKCP-registered psychotherapist and a BACP-accredited supervisor. She has more than ten years' experience working with eating-disordered clients, both in psychiatric settings and in private practice. After setting up a student counselling service and working in primary care, she now has an independent practice as a psychotherapist, supervisor, trainer and examiner. She is currently honorary secretary of the division of counselling psychology.

John Towler, PGCEA, Dip.Hum. Psych., is a freelance counsellor, supervisor and trainer, primarily working in organisational settings. Trained as a priest, he has worked as director of a counselling service and has been a senior lecturer at a tertiary college. He is a consultant for Humanitas and the University of Surrey at Roehampton. He is currently researching influences of the organisation within supervision.

Val Wosket, PhD, is a BACP accredited counsellor and trainer, and senior lecturer in counselling at the College of Ripon and York St John, where she is co-tutor of the Diploma in Supervision. She is author of *The Therapeutic Use of Self: Counselling Practice, Research and Supervision* (Routledge 1999) and co-author, with Steve Page, of *Supervising the Counsellor: A Cyclical Model* (Routledge 2001).

Subject Index

Author Index

Printed by Amazon Italia Logistica S.r.l.
Torrazza Piemonte (TO), Italy

10638368R00123